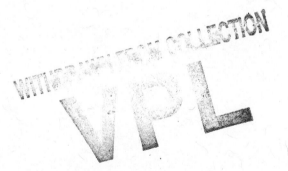

"Angela Hobbs has done it again! Sleep is essential for all of us, and her lucid discussion of factors that can interfere with a good sleep, as well as what can be done to correct the problems, is both easy to read and important information for everyone."

David O. Carpenter, M.D.
Director, Institute for Health & Environment, University at Albany, NY.

***

"...sleep is essential for life and health. To be able to stay awake and to function optimally, one has to have the highest possible quality of one's sleep. It is a fact that more and more people, and especially our young ones, are having severe problems with their sleep, both regarding its depth, quality and length. In Sweden, where I work as a neuroscientist at the prestigious Karolinska Institute, well-known for its Nobel Prize in Physiology or Medicine, more than 1/3 of the entire population has such serious problems, and the percentage seems to increase year-by-year. In other countries the problem is similar, or even worse.

You do not need to agree with all the things that Angela Hobbs says, *Sleep-Powered Wellness* still will give you a lot of food for thought; especially the parts pointing at very simple, easy and cheap suggestions for quick alterations. You may not be able to rid yourself of a lousy boss from one day to another, but you can easily change your bedroom into one that will furnish you with much better conditions to momentarily arrive at the "third pillar of wellness" as Angela Hobbs so elegantly refocuses our thinking. Maybe, however, she should have put it as the "first pillar"; you do realize its enormous importance for your health and your social relationships after you have read this truly thought-provoking, suggestive and mindboggling book.

I strongly recommend it for reading. Now! Before you go to bed tonight.

Professor Olle Johansson,
The Royal Institute of Technology and The Karolinska Institute, Sweden

'Sleep-Powered Wellness' is an invaluable contribution to the health and wellness field. With the escalating pandemic of sleep disorders, many become ensnared by risky long-term medication use to camouflage troubled sleep. In this wonderful book, the author explores and discusses unrecognized causes and factors contributing to sleep problems.

The book is practical, well-written, interesting and provides concrete recommendations for those who are chronically fatigued and debilitated by impaired sleep. Angela systematically describes how to identify major contributors to sleep problems and proposes practical, effective solutions. I look forward to recommending this important book to my patients.

Stephen J. Genuis MD FRCSC DABOG DABEM FAAEM
Clinical Professor, Faculty of Medicine, University of Alberta

***

One of the negative 'hallmarks' of our modern technological age has been a significant increase in insomnia and sleep problems, especially in younger people. Angela Hobbs has managed to go right to the heart of the matter with a practical, very readable and well-researched book that is highly recommended reading for both the public and professionals. This includes people directly impacted by sleep problems, parents concerned about their children's use of wireless devices, doctors and researchers dealing with sleep disorders, and architects in building healthy homes.

Most importantly Hobbs not only examines the many environmental factors that can effect sleep but gives practical solutions to enable the reader to mitigate those factors to achieve what many seek – a healthy and fulfilling night's sleep, night after night.

Don Maisch, PhD. Author of "The Procrustean Approach: Setting Standards for Telecommunications Frequency Electromagnetic Radiation".

***

What a treat to read this extraordinary book! The quality of our sleep is tantamount to the success of our lives - that is a certainty. I live in a world where I speak about the importance of balance, quality sleep, healthy hormones and other wellness principles all day long. In these daily interactions, I see the frustration or even complete ignorance of the general populace when it comes to the health interruptions they encounter daily. Whether chemical assaults, hormone hinderers, poor quality water or even light pollution, most of us are in the dark about the effects on our health. Leave it to a gifted author like Angela Hobbs to bring us into the light. Her latest literary offering is a comprehensive guide on what is making you tired and keeping you awake at night. Not your average book on getting more sleep, this guide will take you to places that will surprise you. She includes lots of opportunity for you to learn new skills for balance and healthy sleep. Entertaining, easy to read, well researched – I learned so much from this book and I know you will too. This book has earned a permanent spot on my office bookshelf. Simply put, an extraordinary book that I am grateful to have read.

Dr. Fiona Lovely B.A. (Adv.), D.C.
Chiropractor, Educator, Women's Health Specialist & Advocate

Also by Angela Hobbs

The Sick House Survival Guide; Simple Steps to Healthier Homes
The Electromagnetic Hypersensitivity Self-Help Workbook
The Sleep-Powered Wellness Self-Help Workbook

Sleep-Powered Wellness

Better Bedrooms for Turbocharged Zzzz's

Angela Hobbs

Bold World Books

Published by:

Bold World Books, a Division of Chinook Solutions Inc.
Calgary, Alberta, Canada
www.chinooksolutions.com

Cataloguing in Publication Data

A catalog for this publication is available from the National Library of Canada

Printed on FSC certified 100% post-consumer recycled paper
Printed and bound in Canada by Transcontinental Printing

Cover design by Chris Hobbs, Alberta College of Art & Design
Manufactured in Canada

First Edition

Table of Contents

Disclaimer

The information in this book is not intended as medical advice, but rather as guidance for identifying and reducing sleep impediments in the bedroom. Always consult your doctor or a knowledgeable medical professional about your symptoms. While every care has been taken to ensure the accuracy of the information, neither the publisher nor the author can accept liability for any errors and omissions.

Acknowledgements

In my first book, *The Sick House Survival Guide; Simple Steps to Healthy Homes,* published in 2003, I told of my recovery from a debilitating encounter with environmental sensitivities and electromagnetic hypersensitivity. My story spawned queries from all over the world. Some were simple, like the one from the man in Mauritius with a mold problem. Some were well beyond my scope, like the woman who'd sprayed her bedroom with insecticide after seeing an ant and then found herself unable to use it. The best I could do for her was to suggest she call the poison control centre, stay out of the bedroom, and shut the door. Most of the queries had some element of sleep disruption — like the husband who couldn't sleep at home but slept well away from home, the wife who developed migraines whenever she slept with the air conditioner working, the son whose grades dropped when the computer and wireless internet were moved into his bedroom.

These queries often required a trip to the medical library; I wanted to be sure that the answers I gave were as up-to-date, accurate, and usable as they could possibly be. That research led me on what initially seemed like disparate paths. One day, I'd be looking for the environmental link to attention deficit disorder; the next week, migraine. A week later, I'd be trying to understand the environmental connection to arthritis; the next, psoriasis. Over time, what initially seemed like unrelated queries began to form a pattern – one related to poor quality sleep, one with very simple and effective solutions.

I'd like to thank everyone who sent me queries; you led me on a learning curve second to none. Everything I learned from working with you forms the core of this book and I'm sure you'll recognize portions of your situations in the cameos.

None of you would have been able to get hold of me without the website and phone tracking provided by Dave Snell, Tim Motz and the talented techies at Ivrnet Inc. Nor would you have wanted to read this book without Jen Groundwater's meticulous editing.

Several medical professionals encouraged my interest in the contribution location can make to our health. My special thanks to Dr. Stephen Genuis, and Dr. June Irwin.

Thanks also to my sons, Christopher and Richard: to Chris for turning my wordy descriptions into illustrations, to Richard for turning them into the "Mistake Meter". Thanks for always being so interested and tolerating the intolerable - A mum with two careers!

An enormous thank-you to my husband Lawrence. What you refer to as my "passion for other people's bedrooms" wouldn't have evolved without your support. You've been there through all the little shuffles and big strides, the wrong turns and the right ones, encouraging me all the way. You could so easily have been jealous, demeaning, and dismissive as this interest ate into more and more of my time. Instead, you've been a true companion, digging deep into your air traffic background to straighten out my understanding of the electromagnetic spectrum and the movement of all those waves. Thank you for being you and for being there.

Thanks to my models, Sunny and Simran Joshi, Sandeep and Sandy Biant, Ross Shephard, and Geoff Genge for featuring in the many pictures that bring so much life to the pages. A special thanks to Sunny for letting Mom take an "upset" picture when you probably just needed a big hug.

Thanks to everyone at Chinook Solutions. You've given me space when I've been torn between two worlds — one seeking a path away from nature, the other a path towards it. Working with you has taught me so much about a strategy's role in navigating turbulence. Your "strategic thinking" has permeated my own thinking and has played a huge part in developing the focus, clarity, definition, and cohesiveness of this book.

Angela Hobbs
Calgary, Alberta
January 2011

Dedication

To all of you who inspired my research-powered journey

Introduction — Sleep Quantity & Quality Both Matter!

Safe, Luxurious Bedrooms and Very Poor Sleep

Whether you're struggling with insomnia, depression, weight gain, migraine or a myriad of other common conditions, your bedroom should be the first, not the last place you look for answers. Our safe, luxurious bedrooms are becoming increasingly difficult to sleep in and are contributing to a range of health issues. This book explains why.

A lot is known about sleep, so you won't find anything new here about the sleep mechanism and the hormones that control it. That part is old hat. Doctors and patients have been toying with that mechanism for years. They've exploited everything from melatonin supplements and herbal teas to relaxation techniques and sleep hygiene. They've adjusted the quantities and timing of glucocorticoid therapies and pain medications, hoping to eliminate the sleep/wake conflict provoked by modern living.

What is new is the approach to tackling that same sleep/wake conflict in the context of the bedroom — the location where that conflict takes place. To some extent we've already recognized the role played by location. When the night closes in, most of us seek out quiet, dark spaces. But as you're about to find out, there are a whole lot more location-specific conditions provoking the sleep/wake conflict than light and noise: microwaves, electricity, contact chemicals, and air pollutants are equally responsible.

You may already have noticed that there are places where you sleep better. These "sleep well, feel well" conditions are often associated with low-stress holidays: the seaside, the lake, the mountains, or the countryside. You may even have tried to recreate those conditions at home — only you couldn't quite put your finger on what it was that made that holiday location so comfortable. Without that crucial piece of information, it's highly likely that your improvements actually took your bedroom further from, rather than closer to, the "sleep well, feel well" conditions you were after.

Like many sleepless others who struggle with the repercussions of fatigue on their demeanour, families, productivity, and health, you may have spent a small fortune on therapies promising to resolve insomnia. You may have endured rigorous measurements at a sleep clinic, or tried energy healing techniques like acupuncture, acupressure and re-resonancing therapies. You may even have found relief in sleep hygiene, massage, or chiropractic manipulation.

If you've tried therapies, you're probably wondering why you keep having to go back — surely once a problem is fixed, it should stay fixed. Yes, it should, but right now, if your bedroom conditions are wrong, any therapy you choose is swimming against a very strong current. An hour of therapy can make very limited progress if the remaining 167 hours of the week are spent in all the wrong conditions. In all likelihood, once you've made some minor bedroom adjustments, your therapy will become progressive. Each visit will build on the success of the previous visit, and your therapist won't have to start from scratch every time.

While not all sleep problems are location-specific, many are. If you've ever noticed that you sleep better in some places and worse in others, there's a good chance that you'll find answers in this book. You spend close to a third of your life in your bedroom — a time crucial to sleep, healing, and intelligence — so getting it right should be the very first step in any effort you make to improve your sleep or health.

Adapting to Changing Bedrooms

Our sleeping and living conditions have undergone tremendous changes since mankind began its transition from being a rural species to being urban. When the transition started in the 1900s, the world's population was about one and a half billion and cities were small. Their size was restricted by the distance a horse could travel and the tolerance people had for the deafening clippity-clop of hooves, the stench of gallons of urine washing down the streets, and the disease inherent in the ever-billowing horse manure and flies. Cities began to grow when sanitation and sewage systems allowed more people to live close together. Those cities grew even bigger when the internal combustion engine and electric power arrived on the scene. Manufacturing and job opportunities increased and it became much easier for people to travel and to live further from their workplace. By 2007, the world's population had reached six billion and half of it had moved into towns and cities; our transition from rural beings to an urban species was complete.

Despite the huge changes that accompanied, and facilitated, that transition, we've made few adjustments to the toolkit we use to navigate them — and this leaves us extremely vulnerable to illness and disease. Our toolkit lags so far behind the developments of the last sixty years that we may even be working on the wrong things in our efforts to gain and maintain health. Many of us put a good deal more effort into selecting the fruit and vegetables that may reduce our cancer risk by four percent[1] than we do into achieving the good sleep that may reduce it by 50 percent.[2] Most of us are far more concerned about the plastics migrating from our water bottles than about the plastics migrating from our pyjamas through the night. We're far more anxious about what goes into our mouths (which passes through a whole detoxification process) than we are about what enters our systems through our lungs and skin (which doesn't get detoxified). Neither the way we define our environment, nor the way we respond to poor health as a result of all those changes is doing us any favours.

Outdated Definition

Much of the time we work with a very traditional definition of our environment, one that doesn't include any of the changes people have made to their surroundings. When the World Health Organization (WHO) assessed the environmental burden of disease in 2006, it used "unsafe drinking water, sanitation and hygiene," "indoor air pollution from solid fuel use," and "outdoor air pollution" as its parameters. With that traditional definition, it estimated that an average of 24 percent of the global disease burden is preventable — in both undeveloped and developed countries. That translates to a cost to Canadians of between $3.6 and $9.1 billion every year.[3] In America, with its much bigger population, those numbers would be about ten times higher.

Had the WHO used a less traditional definition, one that took into account the many new sources of hormonal disruption so fundamental to disease — like infrasound, microwaves and migrating chemicals — it would have discovered much bigger, and more accurate, numbers.

3

Environmental Exposure Effects	Annual Magnitude (Canada)
Deaths	10,000 — 25,000
Hospitalizations	78,000 — 194,000
Time spent in hospital	600,000 -1.5 million days
Restricted activity due to asthma	1.2 -1.8 million days
Cancer	8,000 — 24,000 new cases
Low birth weight babies	500 – 2,500
Total cost	$3.6 — $9.1 billion

How much bigger would these numbers be if we considered the real twenty-first-century environment?

By not recognizing the changes we've made to our environment, we prevent the statistics from reaching the magnitude that would sound alarm bells, threaten certain key industries, question our exploitation of natural resources, and maybe even imperil the economy itself. But in the longer term, trying to ignore our new surroundings is likely to affect the economy just as much. Productivity will drop and health care costs will soar in an intensifying battle against insomnia, depression, stress, absenteeism, diabetes, cancer, immune disorders, and osteoporosis.

Outdated Health Pillars

Since we as a society have not really recognized the health impact of the changes we've made to our environment, we haven't adapted the health pillars with which we navigate it. But diet and exercise, the health pillars we use today, were built during the 1930s when there were fewer chemicals, cars, or synthetic surfaces, little electrical equipment, and no microwaves. The pillars were established by researchers seeking solutions to the health issues presented by a very different environment to the one we live and sleep in today.

Diet and exercise have become enshrined as the major pillars of health to reduce the risk and complications of disease, while sleep has never dominated mainstream conversations about health in the same way. As our environment continues to change, many new diseases and conditions have emerged, and diseases such as cancer have grown increasingly common. Rather than trying to identify why our two main health pillars are ineffective tools in our battle against illness, we've simply shored them up with products and pharmaceuticals.

4

A False Third Health Pillar — Products & Pharmaceuticals

To some extent, products and pharmaceuticals have become our third health pillar. They were quick to usurp the growing void left by inadequate health pillars that considered sleep to be little more than a period of oblivion. Organic foods, dietary supplements, and health club memberships eagerly obliterated our limited understanding. Antioxidants promote health? We're sold! But no one told us that nutritional antioxidants were too short-lived, and too big, to be of any use through the night. Exercise is essential to health? We'll exercise! But no one told us that our weekly 150 minutes of exercise could do us much more good if it was better timed to support the fall of our stress hormones, preventing them from festering through the night.

A Genuine Third Health Pillar — Sleep

Unfortunately, no amount of products, pharmaceuticals, therapies, or supplements can fill the gaps left by inadequate and poor quality sleep. They may make it easier to fall asleep or disguise the symptoms, they may even make those seven to nine hours of oblivion achievable, but if the sleep impediment is right there in the bedroom, drugs and supplements won't give you the quality sleep that you need to be healthy.

To fill these gaps we first have to recognize them. "Do you sleep well?" seems like a simple enough question, and most people would respond without ever considering the attributes reflective of poor sleep. The answer to the question should take into consideration not just the ease with which you fall asleep, sustain sleep, and awaken from it, but also:

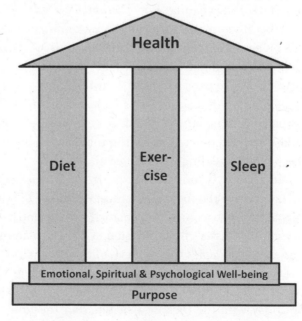

Although 'products' and 'pharmaceuticals' have assumed a dominant role, the third health pillar is actually 'sleep'

- your cravings for all the wrong foods
- your energy level through the day
- your productivity and creativity
- your interest in what's happening around you
- the ease with which you remember
- the speed with which you rise to anger
- the appropriateness of your reactions to the day's many challenges
- the eagerness with which you take on the new day
- the smoothness of your relationships
- the frequency with which you catch colds
- the aches and pains that plague you through the day

If you're not satisfied with how well you measure up to these health indicators, it's time to consider that perhaps you don't sleep well, after all. To deal with these symptoms of poor sleep, you may find that *rather than taking something, you need to take something away*. This book will help you deal with the sleep impediments lurking in your bedroom.

The first chapter, *Sleep Isn't Optional*, describes six important discoveries about sleep and reviews the current understanding of what happens when we're asleep. Far from being a time of nothingness, it's another stage of alertness, one that's crucial to our well-being.

The second chapter, *How Disrupted Sleep Impacts Your Health*, focuses on the importance of strong melatonin and cortisol rhythms. These hormones have roles and responsibilities that extend far beyond initiating and maintaining sleep. Bedrooms that weaken them can contribute significantly to poor sleep and ill health.

Chapter 3 is about *noise*. Here you'll meet Erica and learn of her struggle with noise. We'll look at how noise — both the sounds you hear and those you don't — grew to problematic levels, and why scientists are becoming increasingly concerned about it.

In chapter 4, *microwaves and radio frequency waves* (30 MHz - 300 GHz) become the focus as we meet Alice. We'll look at why these wireless signals have become problematic, why scientists are concerned about them, why Russia's limits are so much lower than ours, and the microwave resonance therapies they've devised to restore sick cells to health.

Chapter 5 introduces *light* and the problems inherent in shift work. We'll look at Edison's light bulb: how it gave us the power to turn night into day with the flick of a switch, and the unforeseen repercussions of that power. The chapter explores the therapeutic uses of light; the health impact of overdosing; and red light's potential to reduce that excess.

In chapter 6, we'll take a look at *household electricity and the earth's magnetic field* and how it disrupted the life of little Stefan. You'll see how the electromagnetic fields created by electricity build up in layers and why scientists are concerned about them. This chapter explores the therapeutic uses of electromagnetic fields, the health impact of the overdose, and our growing understanding of what happens to us when the Earth's magnetic field gets distorted.

Chapter 7 explores the range of *chemicals* that come into contact with your skin as you sleep. You'll see what Chen did to reduce his contact with these chemicals, restore his fertility, and father a child. You'll get an idea of just how far industry will go to protect its products and markets. This chapter looks at our exploitation of the skin's vulnerability for transdermal drug delivery and how that same vulnerability exposes us to an overdose from unbound chemicals in common fabrics and personal care products.

In chapter 8, you'll meet Jenny and witness her struggle with *air pollutants*. Like Jenny, you'll get to see that the very sources that create pollution in our homes are also responsible for impeding its removal. This chapter explores the increasing body of knowledge about the power of ions, and how ionization is being used to reduce infectious bacteria.

Chapter 9 takes you through a worked example of how noise,

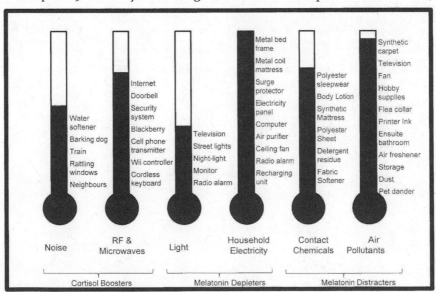

The 'Mistake Meter' prioritizes which conditions you need to tackle first

microwaves, light, electricity, contact chemicals, and air pollutants came together to disturb Mia's sleep. You'll see how she used the Mistake Meter to prioritize the issues she needed to deal with — first in her own bedroom and then in her children's bedroom. In this chapter you'll find instructions for creating your own Mistake Meter and using it to transform your bedroom into one that no longer provokes the sleep/wake conflict.

Chapter 10 considers the importance of reaching beyond our grasp. If the goal of the bedroom is to create a place for healing sleep, then we have to make the informed choices that keep us progressing in that direction.

By the time you get to the end of this book, you'll see your bedroom in a whole different light. You'll understand how conditions in your bedroom are undermining your chances of getting a good night's sleep. You'll know why certain exposures are a greater concern at night than they are during the day — why the wireless transmitter that raises your cortisol by day (when it's already high) doesn't do nearly as much damage as it does when it raises it at night. In other words, from the sleep picture perspective, you don't need to be too concerned about working in a wireless office — just don't sleep in one. You'll understand why the body lotion that depletes your melatonin by night (when it should be high) doesn't do anywhere near the same amount of damage by day. From the healthy sleep perspective, you can apply body lotion liberally during the day — but not at night.

You may find yourself wanting to avoid some exposures altogether, but understanding the exposures in relation to your body clock is the real key. It's a key that allows you to exploit new luxuries and technologies to the full, without paying the price with your health. It's a key that lets you sleep soundly and live well, while still enjoying all that our twenty-first century world has to offer.

Part 1
Sleep, the Third Pillar
of Wellness

1 — Sleep Isn't Optional

Our understanding of sleep and how it evolved

For many people, sleep is a state that's taken for granted. They go to bed, fall asleep, and wake up energized and ready to go about their daily activities. But for others, nighttime is a time of torment. They may feel tired and sleepy before they drag themselves off to bed, but by the time they've completed their ablutions and are tucked up ready for the night, they find themselves wide awake, listening with resentment to the deep slumbering sounds of their families, and fretting about the exhaustion and ineffectiveness that will plague them tomorrow if they don't hurry up and get some sleep. Some of these people will have the added stress that comes from knowing their medical risks increase by 50 percent if they don't get more than five hours of sleep.[1]

In this chapter, we'll take a look at six of the major mid-twentieth-century developments that had to fall into place to reach the current scientific understanding of sleep.

- First, there had to be a shift from the orthodox perception of sleep as a time of nothingness to an acceptance of sleep as a time of considerable brain activity;
- Second, the sleep stages and their activities had to be established;
- Third, melatonin, the hormone that initiates and maintains sleep, had to be discovered;
- Fourth, cortisol's capacity to disturb sleep had to be recognized;
- Fifth, chronobiologists had to determine the drivers of the circadian rhythm;
- And, finally, melatonin's many capabilities and singular role as a healer had to be recognized.

Sleep Recognized — a State of Alertness

The first development came in the form of a shift in the orthodox perception of sleep. For many years seen as a time of nothingness, in 1953 sleep began to be understood as a time of alertness. That shift came when Nathaniel Kleitman and Eugene Aserinsky first discovered and then dramatically demonstrated the eye movements occurring during sleep. Their presentations — using sleeping volunteers — left even previous skeptics in no doubt that the brain's activities continued during sleep. Thanks to this discovery, sleep became recognized as one of four states of arousal.[2]

Sleep is one of four arousal states. The brain is as active during later sleep, sorting and filing away memories, as it is during the day. The system that fuels this activity takes a well-deserved break during the early part of the night. Woe betide anyone who interferes with this replenishing break!

Photo:
Nicola Gilbert

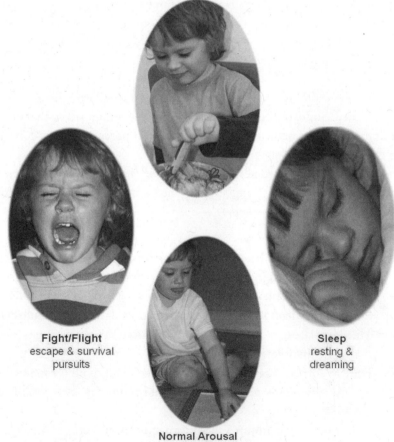

Focused Attention
productive & routine activities

Fight/Flight
escape & survival pursuits

Sleep
resting & dreaming

Normal Arousal
problem-solving & creativity

Sleep Stages Identified

The second development was the realization that sleep happens in stages, with each stage having a specific activity. As the study of sleep progressed, researchers began to see sleep as a time to coordinate and refresh. The brain catches up on the day's information — organizing thoughts, sorting, sifting and filing away memories and knowledge — while the body catches up on healing, resets its clocks, and prepares to take on the new day. All that maintenance takes place as we smoothly and predictably cycle through five sleep stages:

Stage 1 – In this short first phase, all the muscle activity and eye movements begin to slow down. It's easy to wake a person up, but he'll be convinced that he wasn't asleep, regardless of the sleep sounds you may have witnessed. It can be a troublesome stage to get into, especially if late-night activities demand a heightened state of alertness right up to the last minute.

Stage 2 – In a good environment, most people slip seamlessly from Stage 1 into Stage 2 sleep. This much longer second stage is hugely important: we enter the other sleep stages from it and land back in it when they come to an end. Adults spend 45 to 60 percent of the night in this stage in chunks of varying durations.

Stages 3 and 4 – Slow Wave Sleep (SWS). These are the deep sleep stages when it can be incredibly difficult to wake someone up. During Stages 3 and 4, the body uses the day's largest spurt of growth hormone to repair itself and grow. Most of that repair and growth work is completed during the first two or three cycles of the night, leaving more time for Stage 5 during the later part of the night.

Stage 5 – Rapid Eye Movement (REM) sleep. In this dream stage, arm and leg muscles are paralyzed to prevent us from running away with our dreams and getting hurt. As active during this stage as it is during the day, the brain sorts through thoughts, memories, and knowledge and files them away.

A healthy person sleeping in a healthy location passes through five or six complete cycles lasting about 90 minutes each. Assuming there are no bathroom trips or sudden awakenings, the progression of the sleep stages through the night looks something like this:

1-(2-3-4-5-4-3)-(2-3-4-5-4-3)-(2-3-4-5-4-3)-(2-5-2)-(5-2)-(5-2)-1

A Healthy Sleep Stage Sequence

Healing and rejuvenation predominate during the early part of the night, when we have more Stage 4 sleep. During the later hours of the night, stages 5 and 2 share space, giving ample time for filing and storing information so that it can be easily retrieved.

Melatonin Discovered — a Nighttime Antioxidant

The third development was the discovery of melatonin by Aaron Lerner, who was fascinated by the way a tadpole's skin transformed when he fed it pineal glands. Over a period of about four years, he and his team worked their way through some 250,000[3] pineal glands trying to understand what it was about them that changed a tadpole's skin so dramatically. Week after week, the local processing plant delivered clear bags bulging with pineal glands to Lerner's basement laboratory. Here his entourage of excited scientists would cart the bags down the stairs, divvy them up, and settle into their next set of experiments. Lerner finally found the hormone responsible — melatonin — in 1958.[4]

Cortisol Recognized — Stress, both Good and Bad

The fourth development was the recognition of cortisol (glucocorticoids) and the stress response system that Hans Selye had discovered. He wanted to understand how ovaries that hadn't been exposed to chemicals could become diseased. At the time he believed he was on the verge of discovering a new sex hormone, and was surprised to find that he could recreate the lumps and bumps in the ovaries by putting his small furry lab creatures through some pretty stressful situations. For most of these creatures his realization — that both good and bad stress provoke the same response — came too late.

"If the bear doesn't get me, the cortisol will!"

An accumulation of cortisol (stress) kills salmon after spawning

***Photo:** iStockphoto*

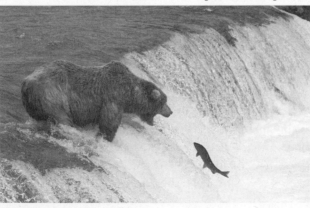

Although Selye discovered cortisol and the stress response system in 1939, it wasn't until chronobiologists started looking for the drivers behind the circadian rhythm that his discovery gained recognition. During much of his career, his peers dismissed his efforts as a waste of time, the pursuit of "meaningless side effects of disease."[5]

Chronobiology Established — the Space Race

The discovery of melatonin and cortisol came into their own when chronobiology became an established science and chronobiologists began looking for the drivers behind the circadian rhythm.

This fifth development was tied up with Russia's launch of Sputnik in 1957, an event that spurred America into addressing the hurdles to manned Mars flights. One of the biggest conundrums was how to handle the weight and space demands of six months' worth of food. Could it be solved by artificially "hibernating" the astronauts?[6]

In the 1950s and 1960s, far more was known about plant rhythms than about human rhythms. But one scientist, Jürgen Aschoff, was deeply interested in human temperature rhythms. He'd even studied his own temperature rhythm in out-of-the-way places like caves where external time cues wouldn't interfere — until he realized that their strong magnetic fields caused their own interference.

When NASA approached Aschoff about its hibernation challenge, he welcomed the opportunity to custom-build a facility in Andechs, Bavaria, where circadian rhythms could be studied without interference from the earth's magnetic field[7] and external time cues. Over the next few years, a host of graduate students took advantage of the facility's solitude to complete their theses while he studied their circadian rhythms in the purity of soundproof, lightproof, temperature-controlled Faraday cages.[8]

Ultimately Aschoff made little progress on the human hibernation front, but he was able to confirm melatonin's role in regulating the body clock, its sensitivity to the earth's magnetic fields, and its potential as a treatment for "rocket-lag." The Andechs facility soon became something of a "chronobiologists' mecca,"[9] attracting scientists from all over the world and establishing chronobiology as a science. Here the natural, unimpeded cortisol and melatonin rhythms that control sleep could be traced. Scientists could see subjects' melatonin rising in the evening, peaking early in the night, and sustaining high levels until early morning, when it dropped to undetectable levels and remained there throughout the day. They could see cortisol dropping through the late afternoon, reaching its lowest point early in the night and beginning its rise during the early morning hours to peak around the middle of the day. Tracing the routine rise and fall of these two hormones contributed significantly to our understanding of the sleep mechanisms.

The routine rise and fall of melatonin & cortisol is essential to quality sleep and vibrant health

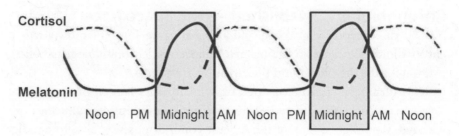

Melatonin's Capacity Uncovered — the Cold War

In 1993, the final piece of the puzzle fell into place when a greater understanding was achieved of the part played by melatonin and cortisol rhythms in initiating and maintaining sleep and wakefulness.

Much of the interest in melatonin came as a result of research provoked by the ongoing hostility between west and east in the aftermath of the Second World War. In the late 1950s and 1960s, the Cold War was intensifying and America feared the hostilities could escalate into a full nuclear war at any time. In anticipation the government increased the funding for research into radiation poisoning treatments. The candidate selected to lead that research was Russel Reiter

Reiter had devoted his career to exploring melatonin, particularly its abundance in active healthy cells and scarcity in sick cells. Exploring answers to this question in the context of radiation poisoning was right up his alley. By 1993, Reiter had discovered that melatonin was abundant in healthy cells because nothing was using it up. It was scarce in unhealthy cells because it was all used up keeping the cell alive. With that question answered, Reiter was able to confirm that the melatonin produced within a person's own body could stabilize the free radicals created by radiation poisoning, and that synthetic melatonin was an ineffective substitute.[10]

Reiter's research provided several starting points for melatonin research that would ultimately lead to a better understanding of the mechanisms controlling sleep.

Completing the Puzzle

Towards the end of the twentieth century, these six discoveries converged to form today's knowledge about sleep. The figure below illustrates how they fit together. Once sleep was established as a subject worthy of study, the sleep stages with their various activities were defined. Combining that with the chronobiologists' discoveries shed light on the roles that hormones play in each of the sleep stage activities.

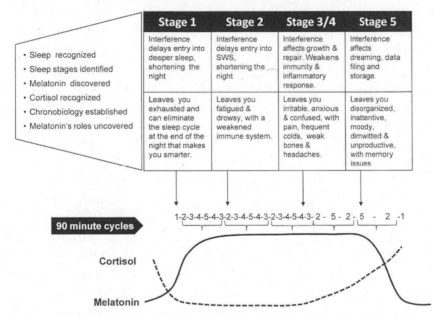

	Stage 1	Stage 2	Stage 3/4	Stage 5
	Interference delays entry into deeper sleep, shortening the night	Interference delays entry into SWS, shortening the night	Interference affects growth & repair. Weakens immunity & inflammatory response.	Interference affects dreaming, data filing and storage.
	Leaves you exhausted and can eliminate the sleep cycle at the end of the night that makes you smarter.	Leaves you fatigued & drowsy, with a weakened immune system.	Leaves you irritable, anxious & confused, with pain, frequent colds, weak bones & headaches.	Leaves you disorganized, inattentive, moody, dimwitted & unproductive, with memory issues

- Sleep recognized
- Sleep stages identified
- Melatonin discovered
- Cortisol recognized
- Chronobiology established
- Melatonin's roles uncovered

90 minute cycles

1-2-3-4-5-4-3-2-3-4-5-4-3-2-3-4-5-4-3- 2 - 5 - 2 - 5 - 2 -1

Cortisol

Melatonin

Current understanding of sleep and the impact of disruption

As more was discovered about melatonin's and cortisol's rhythms, roles, and responsibilities, it became possible to match specific symptoms of sleep deprivation with specific hormone disruptions occurring through the night. Pain on awakening is related to a disturbed cortisol rhythm early in the night, frequent colds are associated with melatonin depletion throughout the night, difficulties falling asleep or awakening are related to a delayed crossover of the two hormones, and so on. With that knowledge, doctors can be very specific about the portion of the sleep curves they target with their therapies and medications.

Good Nights of Bad Sleep & Bad Nights of Good Sleep

Despite all the knowledge we have about sleep today, we're far more adept at recognizing and dealing with sleep disturbances that wake us up than with those that don't. Sleep disturbances that wake us usually speed the heart rate up by 30 beats a minute, while those that only speed the heart rate up by nine beats a minute tend not to wake us up.[11] **But they disturb our sleep just as much**.

The speeded heart rate is initiated when the nervous system picks up on signals in its surroundings. It's a system that would form an extremely sensitive antenna, 27 miles long, if we laid out its cells end to end. It interprets environmental signals as "warnings" (requiring response) or "safety" (requiring no response), and the body adjusts accordingly. Sleep simply can't happen as long as the nervous system is picking up on warnings of danger — we're not designed that way. But those warnings don't necessarily wake us up completely; they can just keep us in an anticipatory mode, preventing us from falling into our deepest and most restorative sleep.

People kept in this anticipatory mode often claim they've achieved seven to nine hours of oblivion. They seldom consider that sleep disturbances may be at the bottom of the symptoms they're experiencing — things like depression, obesity, difficulties coping with the day's challenges, persistent fatigue, difficulty awakening in the morning, recurrent headaches and pain. By not associating their symptoms with disturbed sleep, these people are more likely to continue to achieve the poor sleep quality that makes them more vulnerable to a range of diseases.

A Good Night of Good Sleep

A good night of good sleep is the desirable state. Here the hormone curves cross over twice — once at night when putting us to sleep, and once in the morning when waking us up. The bedroom is free of warning signals and sleep lasts anywhere from seven to nine hours. The sleeper wakes up feeling refreshed and eager to take on the day, and enjoys good health.

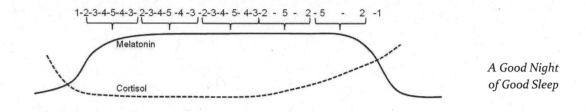

1-2-3-4-5-4-3- 2-3-4-5 -4 -3 -2-3-4- 5- 4-3-2 - 5 - 2-5 - 2 -1

Melatonin

Cortisol

A Good Night of Good Sleep

A Bad Night of Good Sleep

A bad night of good sleep is less desirable. The bedroom is still free of warning signals and there are still only two crossover points — but we awaken before the second one, before all the sleep cycles have completed. The final sleep cycle that makes information retrieval efficient is missed, and because the awakening occurs before the second crossover it can take much longer to really wake up.

Bad nights of good sleep are common among teenagers, people who persist with concentration-demanding activities right up until the moment they drop into bed, and others who turn in for the night still stressed from the day's demands. They lose valuable sleep time waiting for their cortisol levels to drop — a drop that can often be sped up by preserving the last hour of the evening as a time for relaxing activities and gentle exercise. These shorter nights can leave people, and especially teenagers, extremely difficult to deal with, struggling in school, and dissatisfied with themselves.

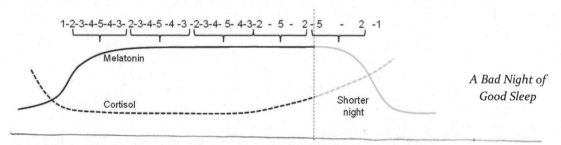

1-2-3-4-5-4-3- 2-3-4-5 -4 -3 -2-3-4- 5- 4-3-2 - 5 - 2-5 - 2 -1

Melatonin

Cortisol

Shorter night

A Bad Night of Good Sleep

A Good Night of Bad Sleep

A good night of bad sleep lasts for long enough, and still has the morning and evening crossovers, but persistent warning signals keep the body in anticipatory mode, ready to respond to danger. A sudden noise or microwave signal will jolt the cortisol curve out of its rhythm. A flash of light or burst of electricity will jiggle melatonin's smooth progression.

Good nights of bad sleep are common among people who live within 300 metres of cell phone transmitters or sleep in brightly lit, noisy conditions where electromagnetic fields and chemicals are plentiful.

A Good Night
of Bad Sleep

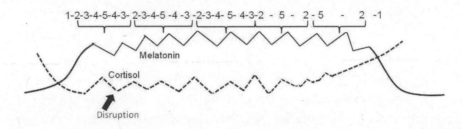

A Bad Night of Bad Sleep

A bad night of bad sleep is the least desirable situation. It combines everything we don't want. The shortened night eliminates the final sleep stage, the morning crossover comes after we wake up, delaying awakening; and endless warning signals keep the sleeper in anticipatory mode ready to respond to danger.

Bad nights of bad sleep are common among flight crews and shift workers. The regularity with which they experience bad nights of bad sleep is associated with their significantly higher risks of cancers and circulatory diseases. Even the World Health Organization recognizes how bad this pattern can be. In 2007, it classified shift work as a probable carcinogen. Bad nights of bad sleep are also common among people who stay awake late into the night, and then try to sleep in locations with abundant sleep disruptors.

A Bad Night of
Bad Sleep

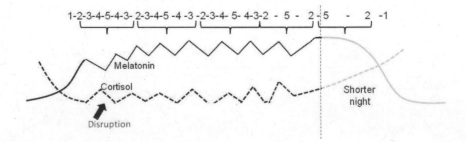

Fig. 1 – The Health Impact of Poor Sleep[12]

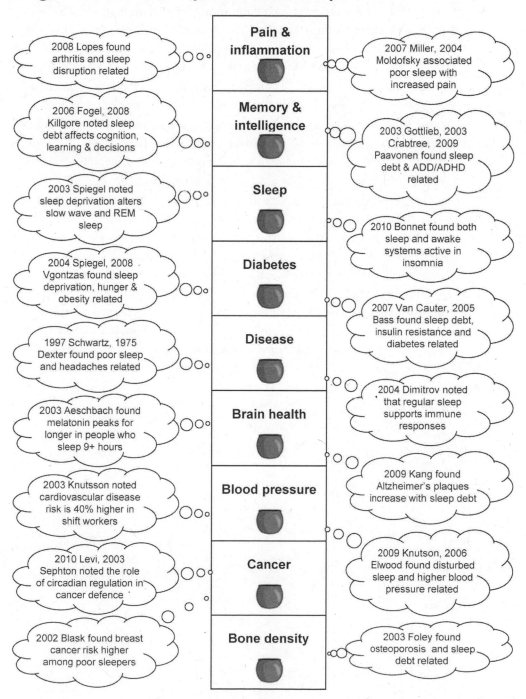

2008 Lopes found arthritis and sleep disruption related

2007 Miller, 2004 Moldofsky associated poor sleep with increased pain

Pain & inflammation

2006 Fogel, 2008 Killgore noted sleep debt affects cognition, learning & decisions

2003 Gottlieb, 2003 Crabtree, 2009 Paavonen found sleep debt & ADD/ADHD related

Memory & intelligence

2003 Spiegel noted sleep deprivation alters slow wave and REM sleep

Sleep

2010 Bonnet found both sleep and awake systems active in insomnia

2004 Spiegel, 2008 Vgontzas found sleep deprivation, hunger & obesity related

Diabetes

2007 Van Cauter, 2005 Bass found sleep debt, insulin resistance and diabetes related

1997 Schwartz, 1975 Dexter found poor sleep and headaches related

Disease

2004 Dimitrov noted that regular sleep supports immune responses

2003 Aeschbach found melatonin peaks for longer in people who sleep 9+ hours

Brain health

2009 Kang found Altzheimer's plaques increase with sleep debt

2003 Knutsson noted cardiovascular disease risk is 40% higher in shift workers

Blood pressure

2009 Knutson, 2006 Elwood found disturbed sleep and higher blood pressure related

2010 Levi, 2003 Sephton noted the role of circadian regulation in cancer defence

Cancer

2002 Blask found breast cancer risk higher among poor sleepers

Bone density

2003 Foley found osteoporosis and sleep debt related

Summary

In the last sixty years, we've come a long way in understanding sleep. The journey began with growing recognition of sleep as a stage of alertness, a shift from previous orthodox thinking that both inspired new discoveries and contextualized others. The sleep picture that evolved allowed doctors to hone in on the specific disturbances related to predictable symptoms and conditions. But the general public just isn't as aware as it could be about the contribution good sleep makes to preventing health problems. Scientists know about how sleep affects us, but our efforts to incorporate good sleep into our daily lives remain limited. Fixing poor sleep should be the starting point in our pursuit of health. Make your sleeping space as healthy as it can be, and then go from there. This book will show you how.

Most of the time, the pursuit of oblivion supersedes the pursuit of quality sleep. As we strive to achieve that oblivion we look to comfort: the mattress, the pillow, the temperature, supplements. That quest has given rise to a $20 billion sleep industry that's having little impact on the $30 billion problem faced by America every year in sleep-related absenteeism, presenteeism, accidents and errors.[13] Our focus on oblivion cheats us of quality sleep, it cheats us of all the health information that accompanies recognized bad sleep, and it cheats us of our health as unrecognized bad sleep situations continue unresolved.

2 — How Disrupted Sleep Impacts Your Health

A tale of two hormones

The sleep and awake systems aren't supposed to be active at the same time. When they are, they become antagonistic: each one prevents the other from fulfilling the functions necessary to keep us healthy. That antagonism sets the scene for a multitude of unpleasant symptoms. This chapter begins by illustrating the sleep/wake conflict with a story of two chefs, one who should only be working at night, the other during the day. It goes on to look at some of the health repercussions that are likely to appear if the conditions provoking the conflict aren't resolved.

The Story of Two Chefs

It was a Saturday night and Chef Melatonin's patience had just about run out. He'd turned up for work every night this week, ready to face the night's jobs, only to find the kitchen a mess. Pots were dirty, beaters were broken, the garbage was full, and the sinks were stained. He could tell this was going to be another night of madness. Tuesday night's soufflé had barely passed as a pancake. Wednesday's salad rolls were covered in crusty black spots and Thursday's creamed soup was lumpy. He dreaded the prospect that the weekend's chocolate fondue was about to turn into a disgusting lumpy brown gravy — but what was he to do? Conditions in the kitchen were deplorable; they'd slipped from the pristine high standards that had lured him to take the position to the shoddy, strained conditions in which he now found himself.

Hoping to make the best of a bad job, he started the night by emptying the overflowing garbage, wiping down the dirty counter, and rewashing the pots until the stubborn, dried-on remains were gone. Already concerned that he wouldn't have time to finish the fondue, he made a start. As he measured the cocoa into the pan, he noticed lumps. He would need to sift and re-measure it. He reached for the syrup, but there was barely enough left in the bottle. He'd have to improvise. As Chef Melatonin turned on the stove, Chef Cortisol appeared through the swinging doors — another fleeting, impromptu visit from the chef who

Constant interference leaves tasks unfinished

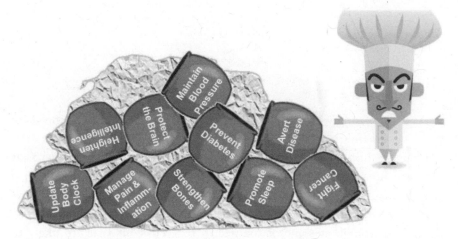

worked the day shift. Chef Cortisol sauntered over, curious about the fondue. It wasn't boiling yet, so he turned up the heat. Unaware of Chef Cortisol's action, Chef Melatonin continued to stir his fondue, expecting a gentle heat to dissolve the fondue's first ingredients, only to find a sudden burst of heat and caramelizing sugar.

Chef Melatonin sat down, his head in his hands. He would have to rethink the recipe with the ingredients available in the pantry, he would have to pray that Chef Cortisol wouldn't make any more unexpected appearances, and he would have to hope that there wouldn't be any more interference thwarting his progress during the remainder of his shift. But even given perfect conditions, it was highly unlikely that he would be able to complete the night's work and leave a clean kitchen with the little bit of time left before morning.

On his way home, Chef Melatonin walked past Chef Cortisol seated at a table, thumbing through an untidy stack of recipes. Matches wouldn't have held his eyes open as he searched for that prized scrap of paper — the one on which he'd written the proportions for that moist chocolate cake. Maybe he'd make this mushroom dish, or that corn fritter, maybe this vegetable medley — the distractions came thick and fast and none of his substitutes would augment the dessert tray. Chef Cortisol gathered up his pile of papers and dragged himself toward the kitchen. The garbage was overflowing, the pans were encrusted, and his day began with much the same catch-up as Chef Melatonin's had before him. He reached for the long, sharp knife that would slice right through the breakfast melon; it slipped...

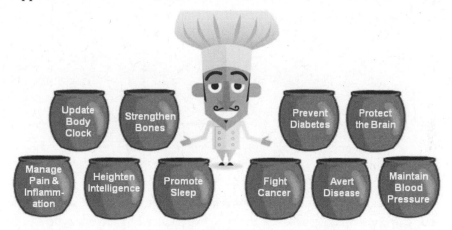

Minimal interference gets tasks finished

The Many Roles of Melatonin and Cortisol

The story illustrates the struggle that melatonin, goes through every night as a result of bedroom mistakes that overload its capacity, deplete its resources, and interfere with its progress. The dirty saucepans, overflowing garbage, and broken beaters represent the burden imposed by unnecessary chemicals, light, and electromagnetic fields. Chef Cortisol has no business being in the kitchen at night. He represents the cortisol that doesn't get to rest at night because of the incessant prodding of things around him. Neither melatonin nor cortisol — can function properly with the amount of interference that surrounds them... and they have an awful lot to do:

Update the Body Clock

Melatonin's primary role is to use light conditions to update the master body clock. Other systems then feed off that update, ensuring that the body's many activities happen at the right time and in the right sequence.

To set that clock, cells in the eye watch for changes in light intensity. When it's light, they signal melatonin production to stop and cortisol production to start, initiating the morning crossover that wakes us up.[1] When it's dark, an absence of signals restarts melatonin production and stops cortisol production,[2] initiating the nightly crossover that makes us fall asleep.

Whenever melatonin levels drop, cortisol levels should rise, and whenever melatonin levels rise, cortisol levels should fall. In a perfect world with no interference, the two hormones should rise and fall predictably and in opposition to each other at dawn and dusk.

Melatonin & cortisol should rise and fall predictably in opposition to each other at dawn and dusk

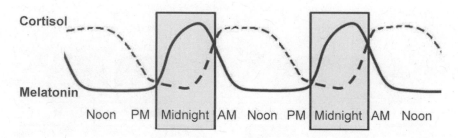

Any interference to these rhythms affects other dependant systems and that can cause major chaos[3] — the type experienced by anyone who's been staying up late, changing shifts, or flying on a plane. Suddenly you're being woken by hunger, shivering in the middle of the day, and highly sensitive to smells as the body's water, temperature, and blood volume systems struggle with the inaccurate time signal. Ultimately, if the chaos persists, the de-synchronization of the body's many systems affects our ability to avoid and recover from illness.[4] When mice experience a similar amount of de-synchronization, they're just as likely to die from it as they are to survive it.

Our appetite-controlling hormones, leptin and ghrelin, depend heavily on an accurate time signal from the body clock.[5] When the clock is accurate, leptin suppresses our appetites at night so that feelings of hunger don't interfere with sleep. Ghrelin stimulates our appetites by day. When the clock's accuracy fails, these appetite regulators get confused, leaving us hungry for all the wrong foods at all the wrong times. It only takes two four-hour nights to increase a person's appetite by 45 percent.[6] People are 73 percent more likely to eat themselves fat[7] if they only get four hours of sleep. That drops to 50 percent if they sleep for five hours and 23 percent if they sleep for six hours.

Hours of sleep	Increased likelihood of obesity
6	23%
5	50%
4	73%

People who sleep less than six hours are more likely to eat themselves fat

Manage Pain and Inflammation

Inflammation is the body's way of isolating, immobilizing, and eliminating pathogens. Melatonin and cortisol both play a role in the inflammation response, with melatonin stimulating it and cortisol resolving it; hence the use of cortisol creams to heal infected sores and glucocorticoid therapies for asthma and lung inflammations. These cortisol medications can make it almost impossible to sleep.

When bedroom conditions weaken the melatonin-cortisol rhythm, the inflammation response gets weaker. The unresolved inflammation of this weakened response can leave a person in pain, performing poorly, and sleepy. It can damage tissue and may contribute to early-morning heart attacks and strokes[8]. It's often at the root of pain conditions, especially the early morning pain that plagues many arthritis sufferers.[9]

Heighten Intelligence

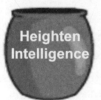

Cortisol is primarily a daytime hormone. It makes its first appearance towards the end of the night when our brains are sorting through information from the previous day and creating strategies for success. As dawn breaks, cortisol levels rise; this rise continues into the early afternoon. Cortisol gives us the alertness and concentration we need to be productive and creative. In the late afternoon, those levels begin to fall again, reaching a nightly low just after sleep consumes us.

This nightly low, or recovery period, is critical to our ability to respond appropriately to the stresses we face during the day, to our creativity, and to our productivity. It's a good time for that break since there should be little demand for alertness, creativity, movement, problem solving, or escape then — at least on a regular basis.

When bedroom conditions interfere with cortisol's nightly rest period, we tend to awaken repeatedly — if we can get to sleep in the first place.

We wake up groggy and spend the day fatigued, inattentive, irritable, quick to anger, and struggling to remember. That's a starting point that makes it difficult to be intelligent, creative or productive.

Promote Sleep

We depend on strong melatonin and cortisol rhythms to sleep soundly. When melatonin reaches its highest levels, it lowers our body temperature and opens the sleep gate. When these rhythms are undisturbed the sleep stages run smoothly and predictably. With a long enough night these rhythms ensure that the sleep cycles are complete. Surrounded by conditions that support the melatonin and cortisol rhythms we awaken rested, refreshed, alert and ready to take on the new day.

When bedroom conditions weaken the rhythm, melatonin doesn't reach the high levels necessary to lower our body temperature or open the sleep gates. So instead of a long night of seamlessly switching sleep stages, we get the intermittent, unpredictable sleep stages that leave us tossing and turning. That's the kind of sleep that's often associated with the weak melatonin rhythm of newborn babies, the elderly, and people suffering from depression, Parkinson's disease, and Alzheimer's disease.[10]

Prevent Diabetes

The stress system that keeps us alert and responsive during the day ensures that there's enough glucose in our bloodstreams and enough insulin available to carry it to our muscles. With all that available energy we can be active and productive. The system counts on seven to nine hours of physical inactivity at night — a period when there's no reason for glucose or insulin to be present.

Bedroom conditions that boost cortisol levels keep us in this alert and responsive state for longer than necessary. The conditions encourage our active periods to eat into our inactive periods. Over time, this can translate into an unnecessary, but almost perpetual, stream of glucose and insulin — a state that contributes to insulin resistance and diabetes. Repeatedly sleeping for less than four hours a night ensures this ongoing presence of glucose. It takes as little as six of these short nights to reduce a person to a pre-diabetic state.[11]

Avert Disease

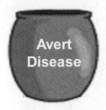

When our cells create the energy they need to go about their various activities, they also produce free radicals. When contained, these molecules play valuable roles in communicating between cells and fighting disease, but when un-contained they become dangerous. Antioxidants contain these molecules by giving them the missing electron they're looking for and bringing what can be quite an aggressive hunt to an end.

During the day, vitamins from our food and supplements provide those antioxidants, but few of them are available at night, and those that are have specific conditions under which they're willing to work. That makes us heavily dependent on melatonin because, unlike dietary antioxidants, it's available and isn't specific about its work conditions.

Much of melatonin's antioxidant activity involves containing nitric oxide levels. Nitric oxide is a free radical that plays a role in communication, blood flow regulation, and as a toxin to kill bacteria and pathogens, but when there's too much of it, it's implicated in asthma, breathing disorders, and heart attacks.

When bedroom conditions interfere, melatonin's capacity to neutralize free radicals can get overwhelmed. When there's not enough melatonin to keep up with the constant flow of free radicals, a situation known as "oxidative stress" occurs. Here the free radicals' hunt for missing electrons gets out of hand, damaging cells, DNA, surrounding tissues, and organs. Oxidative stress contributes to aging and many diseases.

Protect the Brain

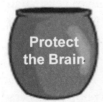

Much of our cellular nighttime activity takes place in our brains. This activity requires copious amounts of energy and results in the production of an abundance of free radicals. The antioxidants necessary to contain these molecules can't be food-sourced because they're too big to penetrate the blood-brain barrier and reach the brain,[12] which is where they're needed. That means we have to depend on melatonin, both because it's small enough to penetrate the barrier and because it stimulates the production of other more specific antioxidants like glutathione.

When bedroom conditions interfere with melatonin and cortisol, our cells become defenceless, deprived of both protection and energy. The interference to melatonin reduces how many specific antioxidants it produces, while the elevated cortisol eats into the antioxidants that melatonin has managed to produce, while also diverting any energy towards the muscles, readying them for action. This reduced protection and confusion sets the stage for the development of cruel neuro-degenerative diseases like Alzheimer's, Parkinson's, and Huntington's diseases, as well as schizophrenia.[13]

Maintain Blood Pressure

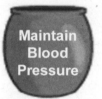

Typically our blood pressure follows the cortisol rhythm, falling as melatonin's antioxidant capacity rises at night, and rising as melatonin's antioxidant capacity wanes in the morning.

When bedroom conditions reduce melatonin and therefore its antioxidant capacity, it struggles to keep the blood pressure down. As a result our circulatory systems get strained and our hearts get weaker. Heart attacks often occur in the early morning hours when melatonin's antioxidant capacity is all used up.[14]

Fight Cancer

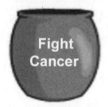

Melatonin is about 40 percent lower in cancer patients than in people who are cancer-free.[15] Abundant melatonin inhibits cancer in several ways: by containing estrogen,[16] preventing mutated cells from becoming malignant tumours,[17] and decreasing telomerase activity.[18] Telomerase is an enzyme in cancer cells, stem cells, and germ cells that lengthens the telomeres — the end caps of chromosomes that dictate how many times a cell can divide. A cell with a longer telomere can multiply more than one with a shorter telomere. So if there's nothing to stop telomerase from lengthening the cell's telomere, the cell will be able to reproduce indefinitely — regardless of whether it's sick or healthy. If it's the sick cells that multiply, cancer can result.

When bedroom conditions push melatonin levels down and cortisol up, keeping our cells healthy becomes a huge challenge. On the one hand, the reduced melatonin leaves telomerase abundant, the telomeres long, and reproduction indefinite — whether the cells are healthy or sick. On the other, the elevated cortisol shortens the telomeres in healthy cells, limiting their reproduction[19]. Interfering with the length of our telomeres is associated with cancer, heart disease, and decreased life expectancy.

Strengthen Bones

Strengthen Bones

We depend on a strong melatonin and cortisol rhythm to make our bones and keep them strong.[20] Melatonin is involved in instigating the day's biggest spurt of growth hormone.

When bedroom conditions weaken the rhythm, the strength and health of our bones suffer. Depleted melatonin levels make it difficult to build up the bones. Higher cortisol levels reduce the amount of calcium that can be absorbed[21] and the amount of growth hormone that's released, ultimately making bones weaker and increasing the risk of injury and osteoporosis. Persistently elevated cortisol is the most common cause of osteoporosis in adults aged 20-45 years. It affects 10 million Americans, while low bone mass affects another 34 million — mostly women. Despite its prevalence, there's been little research into the connection between osteoporosis, reduced bone mass, and disrupted sleep.

Figure 2 shows some of the studies into the roles that melatonin and cortisol play in our sleep and health.

Fig. 2 — The Many Roles of Melatonin & Cortisol[22]

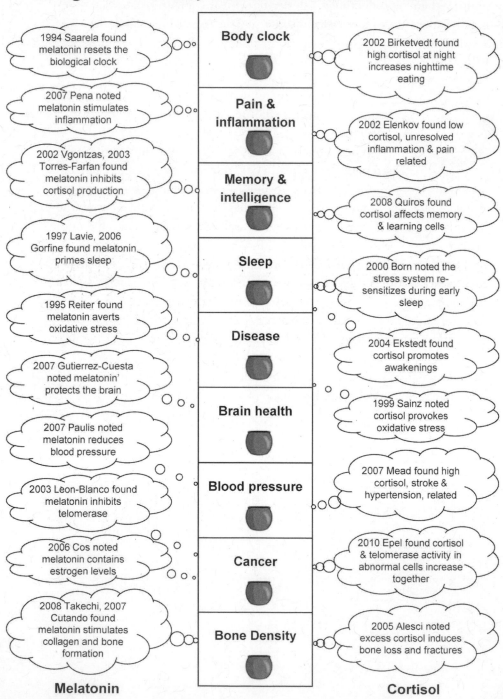

1994 Saarela found melatonin resets the biological clock

2007 Pena noted melatonin stimulates inflammation

2002 Vgontzas, 2003 Torres-Farfan found melatonin inhibits cortisol production

1997 Lavie, 2006 Gorfine found melatonin primes sleep

1995 Reiter found melatonin averts oxidative stress

2007 Gutierrez-Cuesta noted melatonin' protects the brain

2007 Paulis noted melatonin reduces blood pressure

2003 Leon-Blanco found melatonin inhibits telomerase

2006 Cos noted melatonin contains estrogen levels

2008 Takechi, 2007 Cutando found melatonin stimulates collagen and bone formation

Body clock

Pain & inflammation

Memory & intelligence

Sleep

Disease

Brain health

Blood pressure

Cancer

Bone Density

2002 Birketvedt found high cortisol at night increases nighttime eating

2002 Elenkov found low cortisol, unresolved inflammation & pain related

2008 Quiros found cortisol affects memory & learning cells

2000 Born noted the stress system re-sensitizes during early sleep

2004 Ekstedt found cortisol promotes awakenings

1999 Sainz noted cortisol provokes oxidative stress

2007 Mead found high cortisol, stroke & hypertension, related

2010 Epel found cortisol & telomerase activity in abnormal cells increase together

2005 Alesci noted excess cortisol induces bone loss and fractures

Melatonin

Cortisol

Summary

Melatonin and cortisol have a wide array of capabilities and responsibilities. To fulfill these roles, they need our support, not our interference. For peak performance, melatonin needs to rise at night and fall in the morning, while cortisol needs to fall at night and rise in the morning. The quality of our sleep and health depends on these rhythms being strong and predictable with only the occasional bit of interference. When that interference becomes regular, our sleep suffers, symptoms develop, and ultimately illness and disease set in.

Those bedroom mistakes usually involve six groups of exposures: the noise and microwaves that elevate cortisol, the light and electromagnetic fields that deplete melatonin, and the contact chemicals and air pollutants that distract melatonin from doing a thorough job. In the next six chapters we'll look at these six exposures individually.

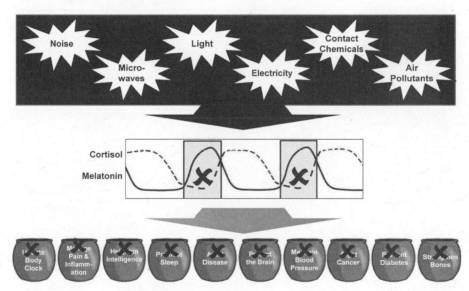

Any of the six factors that disrupt this hormone rhythm raises the risk of developing ten increasingly common conditions

Part 2 — Six Factors That Disrupt & Impede Sleep

3 — Noise and Infrasound

Quieting harmful sounds that may not wake you up

Noise reverberating through our homes can be extremely annoying. It provokes unpleasant symptoms in our bodies, brings us to a state of alertness during the night, and lingers in the hard surfaces that surround us. At night, noises can come from inside by way of appliances, air conditioners, ventilation systems, snoring partners, and entertainment systems. Outside noises can include exaggerated mufflers on cars leaving the pub at two o'clock in the morning, airplanes flying overhead, trains thundering down the tracks, wind turbines, or emergency vehicle sirens. Homes in many medium- and high-density housing developments reverberate as neighbouring garage doors slam closed. Thin common walls leave us exposed to others' family discord, snoring, and the "living" sounds of shift workers with opposing life schedules. In recent decades, there has been growing recognition of noise as a pollutant. It is now being recognized that nighttime noise can provoke the awake system and make us sick. Fortunately, we are also gaining a better idea of how to reduce noise; I'll explore some techniques and materials in this chapter.

We'll tell Erica's story to illustrate the impact night noises can have on our sleep and health. Next we take a look at the development of noise as a pollutant, how it's used therapeutically to restore healthy vibrations to our cells, its impact in overdose quantities, and what can be done to reduce it.

Erica's Story

The broken English coming down the phone line belonged to an older German lady. Suzanne explained that after four years, she had finally made her "trip of a lifetime" to visit her daughter Erica and her grandchildren,

Sam and Marianne. Just a week into her trip, she was concerned about the location of her daughter's house. It was so reminiscent of the Munich community where she'd brought up her own children, right down to the airplanes barreling down the nearby landing strip at all hours of the day and night. Suzanne's biggest worry was Erica's forgetfulness: when they went out shopping together, Erica would forget the most basic things: she would have to ask the salesperson for the price three or four times. At home, this young mother would reprimand her children for doing things she'd given them permission to do just moments earlier.

Erica thought she'd chosen the perfect house in an ideal community. Everything was just a short walk away: the school, the playground, the library, the shops, the doctor's office. The area was flat, safe, and perfect for her children to ride their bikes after school. The only thing that really annoyed her was its proximity to the airport; the planes coming in low would vibrate the knick-knacks and send tremors through the fish tank, but after three years of living here, she'd more or less grown used to it. After all, she had grown up right near the Munich airport before it moved.

Erica had forgotten all about the study that took place in her Munich community when she was young. She hadn't participated in it, though some of her friends had, and she remembered feeling left out as other kids left their classrooms to go with the important-looking visitors.

A new airport opened in Munich in 1992, and before the old one closed down, enterprising scientists set up studies on the effect of noise on primary-school children so they could compare before and after. Those studies found that airplane noise affected the children's motivation and learning. Before the airport moved, the ten-year-olds couldn't have been less interested in solving the myriad of puzzles in front of them. After the airport moved, they became far more engaged. They would try repeatedly to solve puzzles; they improved their grades, and they began aiming higher at school. Subsequent cumulative research shows that for every five decibels that noise repeatedly rises over background levels, a child's reading ability lags by two months.[1]

As her mother reminded her of the studies and what they revealed, Erica became anxious about her children and began to do a bit of research. The more she found out, the more concerned she became. There was so much research connecting noise to a child's reading ability and long-term memory.[2] As she pondered what she'd read, she began to question if maybe the airport noise was responsible for the change in Sam and Marianne's "brightness."

Until their move, Sam and Marianne had been just as smart as her friends' children. They'd been in preschool together, learning to recognize their letters and sounds and proudly reciting their ABC's. However, now as eight- and nine-year-olds, they were struggling to achieve a satisfying level of reading fluency. While her friend's children were chuckling their way through Harry Potter, her own children were still asking her to read it to them.

Erica was pretty confident that her children would ultimately become bookworms like she and her husband were. In the meantime, she quite liked sharing Harry's Quidditch games with them. She was reassured to know that the learning and memory cells killed by her children's persistent noise exposure and subsequent high cortisol levels would ultimately be replaced. She was relieved to hear that their learning problems would reverse[3] once those cortisol levels were restored to their normal rhythm.

What bothered Erica far more than the cognitive connection was the health connection. Could the high noise levels the family was exposed to explain her young husband's recurring headaches and arthritis-type pains? Could it be responsible for her sporadic dizziness, disorientation, and memory issues, and the children's frequent colds? It might even account for the grouchy faces sitting across from her at the breakfast table. If noise could explain the kids' struggle with Harry Potter, could it also explain these other symptoms?

What Erica Did

As we worked through her house, Erica began to see that there were ample opportunities to reduce the amount of noise getting in. She soon got to work and added a third layer of glass to the double-glazed windows in the bedrooms. She took off the inside wooden window trims and filled any gaps before replacing them and sealing the edges with a flexible sealant. Erica added a second storm door to the outer doors at the front and back of her house, and added another layer of insulation in the attic.

With all the weakest sound barriers to her home reinforced, the noise level inside dropped dramatically. But Erica had become very conscious of the sounds that still penetrated and reverberated through her house. To reduce them further, she sealed cracks around pipes and wires, replaced the hollow interior doors with solid ones, placed cork squares between hard surfaces to prevent sound vibrations from moving between them, and positioned homemade sound absorbers in the bedroom corners.

Before long, the faces surrounding Erica at the breakfast table were cheerier and more excited about the day ahead. Erica was less forgetful and her children worried less that she would be angry with them. Her husband's headaches and pains subsided dramatically. Now only the odd plane woke them in the night — enough for Erica and her husband to know that the next step in their life together would be to move to a much quieter location.

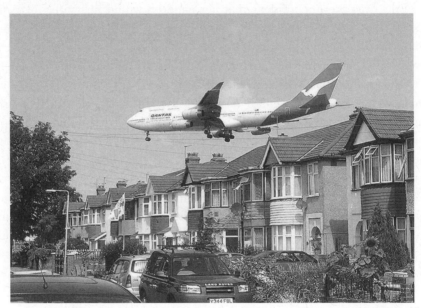

Transportation noise raises cortisol levels, interfering with sleep quality and contributing to disease

Photo:
Adrian Pingstone July 2004

Noise Pollution

Where Did It Come From?

Long before we understood how detrimental noise can be to our health, scientists were curious to understand how it moved from its source to the receiver's ears, how it set the eardrum vibrating, and how it was translated by the brain as sound.

Pythagoras, the Greek scientist, pondered the question at length. He concluded that the widths of the visible blur surrounding an instrument's strings were related to the loudness or softness of the sound. Aristotle expanded on this concept, suggesting that the "blurring" strings were striking air molecules. He showed us that in a vacuum, where there is no air; sound doesn't travel and therefore can't be heard. Vitruvius, who studied echoes and reverberations to build his theatres, went even further, suggesting that sound moves through the air much like waves in water.

When Galileo turned his attention to sound's movement, he added the concept of the "standing wave:" once sound is introduced to a trapped air column, it can only move to and fro along the column. Most instruments are based on the concept of the standing wave. They use the player's lips or a reed to introduce a vibration into the column and then vary the length of the air column to change their sound. String instruments, like an acoustic guitar, create a standing wave on the string by clamping it at both ends. Once the vibrations reach the clamp, they have no alternative but to retrace their steps. As the vibrations travel to and fro, they make the sound box vibrate. The vibrating sound box sends the sound waves out into the surrounding air and to the receiver's ears. This concept of the standing wave becomes important when we begin to look at ways of reducing sound vibrations, and also later when we turn our attention to the movement of electricity and its electromagnetic fields.

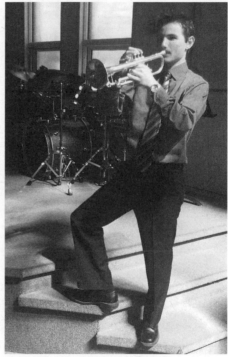

Ross uses his lips to introduce a standing wave to the trumpet's trapped air column. As he changes the size of the column the sound changes

Photo:
Angela Hobbs

During the eighteenth and nineteenth centuries, these early concepts about sound's movement evolved into an understanding of how sound moves through solids, liquids, and gases. By the middle of the twentieth century, we were transmitting sound over long distances — right into living rooms. Families that had once gathered to hear the news in town squares now gathered around the radio. At first we used electrical wires, and later wireless radio frequency waves and microwaves, to deliver sound to distantly located amplifiers. Once the sound was delivered to the amplifier, loudspeakers restored it to its original sound wave and it resumed its journey, travelling through the air to whichever ear happened to be in range.

Where Did It Go?

As sound-moving technologies advanced, broadcasting blossomed and the entertainment industry boomed. The deafening clippity-clop of horses' hooves that had caused so many noise complaints during the nineteenth century was replaced by a whole new set of sounds...and a whole new set of complaints. City dwellers could hear the neighbours' televisions, radios,

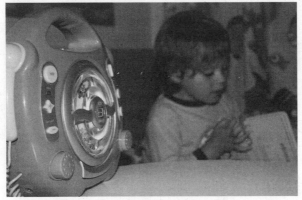

The development of personal sound equipment meant noise could be created anywhere, at any time, and at any volume

Photo:
Nicola Gilbert

and stereos, and they were being awoken by those sounds — sounds over which they had absolutely no control. This absence of control soon proved to be a whole new source of stress.

While transmitted sounds became more of a problem, the sources of noise inside homes proliferated as well. New luxuries and labour-saving devices — washing machines, dryers, dishwashers, water softeners, air conditioners, furnaces, refrigerators — brought a new level of noise right inside.

Ironically, advances in the building industry have made many of these noises much more penetrating and much more difficult to deal with. New building materials and methods remove many of the sound barriers and deflectors that were common in earlier homes. Walls are now less dense and often rely on a metal framework and lightweight thermal insulation; ventilation systems add lengths of hollow metal tubing that propagate sound. Lower-density synthetic furniture, prevalent hardwood floors, and the removal of many noise absorbers like curtains and rugs — whether due to home fashions or allergies — have left many homes with few sound-absorbent surfaces. The result is that bedrooms are now places where sounds penetrate easily from both inside and outside the house, and within which sound vibrations move freely.

The Dose and the Overdose

Dose — Sound as a Therapy

Most of us recognize the impact sound can have on our mood, it can soothe us, perk us up and even make us eat faster — a quality that restaurants often exploit! The ergonomics industry, energy healing techniques, and the healing ceremonies of many indigenous societies are based on the effect that sound and its vibrations has on the body's cells. Few indigenous peoples' healing ceremonies were or are complete without drums, clapping, pulsating, and chanting. One might explain the change in the patient's state on a spiritual level, by saying the sounds "summon spirits" who either return the patient to health or accompany him into the spirit world. A more scientific explanation is that these low-frequency sounds re-resonate the patient's sick and ailing cells, restoring health.

While many of today's energy healing therapies use sounds of the right frequency and volume at the right time to effect healing, few hospital treatments are on-board. In many ways, sterile hospital environments, with their range of unnatural sounds, have foregone the re-resonancing potential of natural sounds. The sounds they're replaced with may even increase the resonance disruption in sick and ailing cells.

Since the middle of the twentieth century, there has been renewed interest in how sound — both audible and inaudible — can contribute to healing. In music therapy, audible sound is used to coordinate the body's internal and very elaborate communication system. People with a poorly coordinated system, like those with autism spectrum disorder or ADHD, often struggle to learn, concentrate, process information, and sometimes even move in a coordinated way. Alfred Tomatis discovered that this internal communication system could be improved using sound. His method has been used successfully to improve learning, concentration, information processing, and movement.

Resonance therapies, including vibration therapy, cymatics, sound wave therapy, and sound bioresonance, are more likely to use inaudible sound. The process is similar to acupuncture, but instead of needles being used to channel energies through the meridians, sound is used. Sound vibrations travel down the meridians to sick cells. When the healthy vibration reaches a sick cell, the latter becomes "re-resonanced" – eventually restoring it to a healthy state and normal functioning.

Overdose — Sound as a Health Risk

The airport findings mentioned above (not only Munich, but also London and Los Angeles moved airports and were the site for similar studies) were accompanied by an increasing number of people suffering from vibroacoustic disease. Traditionally, only aircraft technicians and workers in heavy industry developed the breathing and central nervous system disorders of vibroacoustic disease[4] due to their elevated exposure to sounds in the infrasound and low-frequency range. Infrasound is defined as sound waves with frequencies below the lower limit of human audibility. With the growth of heavy industry, transportation networks, and wind farms, sources of noise in this range have increased dramatically. As a result, larger segments of the population are exposed to noise and even children are being diagnosed with vibroacoustic disease. The US Environmental Protection Agency estimates that about 138 million Americans are exposed to "excessive" noise levels.

Noise is so indubitably a health risk that the World Health Organization has set "night noise" targets of 40 decibels or less; these guidelines fall just below the noise levels associated with more serious and costly health conditions. It also directed cities with over 250,000 residents to produce and use noise maps to target their noise reduction strategies.

The WHO recommends a night noise guideline of 40dB

Decibel	Impact[5]	Sound
0		Threshold of hearing
10		Low whisper
30	Disturbed sleep	Soft music
35	Increased annoyance	
40	More awakenings and sleep enhancing supplements	Dripping faucet
45	Environmental insomnia	Average home
55	Cardiovascular disease, annoyance & sleep disruption	Busy restaurant
60-70	Heart attacks, hypertension	Normal conversation
75-85	Psychological symptoms	Busy traffic
80		Window AC unit
90-115		Screaming child, thunder
120		Ambulance siren
134		Threshold of pain

Infrasound

As cities have grown, transportation networks have broadened, heavy industry has expanded, and people have acclimatized to the twenty-four-hour day, tremendous demands have been made on fossil fuel. These are needed to mine raw materials, produce goods, deliver those goods, and keep them powered. In the last 25 years, all that growth and activity has eaten up as much oil as was consumed in all of previous history combined.[6]

That hearty appetite has fuelled the search for other ways of producing electricity, and the world's current favourite is wind energy.[7] It's interesting, though, to note that there is some debate over the fossil-fuel savings wind energy provides — a two-megawatt turbines like those used in North America's has an impressive list of fossil fuel ingredients.

Ingredients needed to produce a two-megawatt wind turbine:

- 170 tonnes of coking coal
- 300 tonnes of iron ore
- Additional fossil fuels for mining ingredients
- Additional fossil fuels for heating ingredients
- Additional fossil fuels for shipping ingredients
- Additional fossil fuels for transporting final turbine

Without perfect conditions few wind turbines ever produce enough electricity to offset the fossil fuels used to make them

A wind turbine has to sustain its peak performance for three years before it begins to produce more energy than was used to make it — a level of performance that many turbines don't achieve during their entire 25- to 30-year lifespan. Despite the enormous demands they make on our dwindling fossil fuels and the contribution that makes to greenhouse gas emissions, wind farms have become popular amongst energy generators.

Today, Canada is home to 10,000 of North America's 17,000 wind turbines.[8] And the country's unwillingness to observe the setback distances recommended by the World Health Organization has probably contributed to nearby residents' poor sleep and feelings of having spent the night in a washing machine or trapped in an organ pipe.

The World Health Organization recommends a distance "in excess of two kilometres"[9] between turbines and residences. But while the Dutch, with their wealth of windmill experience, have swallowed the additional costs of building their new wind farms out at sea to ensure this distance from residences, North America has settled on a mere half-kilometre setback[10] and added a new dimension of "audibility" to noise assessments: if the noise frequency falls outside our hearing range at normal volumes, then it only becomes a problem if it becomes loud enough to hear.

The problem here is that the infrasound that wind turbines emit falls below the frequencies most people can hear. Animals certainly hear it — it's widely used by elephants, rhinos, tigers, and whales to communicate with each other through dense forests and great oceans. To them infrasound is like a built-in cell phone that, despite their separation by vast distances and thick foliage, ensures male elephants converge on ovulating females, brings them together around the same watering hole, and warns animals of tsunamis and volcanic eruptions, making them run.

But for people to register a sound in the infrasound range, they have to crank up the volume to about 110 dB — that's loud. And even then, they wouldn't actually hear it, they would just sense an intense pressure and vibration. To get an idea of just how loud that is, and how much energy that brings into your bedroom, imagine the loudest music you've ever heard — the rock band that shook the concert hall. Now double it! That's the volume and energy level that infrasound has to reach before North America considers it harmful. People living by wind farms feel this pressure and feeling of vibration all the time, and it's a definite stressor, though there isn't anything they can hear in the ordinary sense; it's all going on at the infrasound level.

Most of our wind farms try to keep the volume below 85 dB, but those daytime measurements, often taken ten feet from the ground, don't reflect the volume at the top of a 100-foot turbine during the evening and night, when air conditions and background noises are very different.

The graph below illustrates the intensity that sounds of different frequencies have to reach before most people are able to hear them. The shaded area to the left of the graph is the infrasound range between 0 and 20 Hz.

The damage that infrasound can do is fortunately recognized enough to prevent wind farms from being built near zoos or wildlife reserves. It's also recognized by the ergonomics industry that designs workstations and tools. This industry follows standards set out by the International Standards Organization[11] (ISO) — standards that recognize the body's

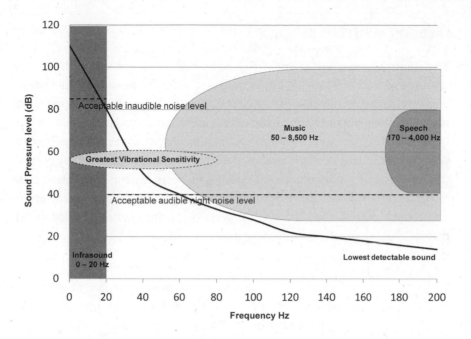

Just how loud, or energized, a sound has to be before we "hear" it depends on its frequency.

Sound doesn't cease to exist just because a deaf person can't hear it.

susceptibility to these frequencies when they become too energized. At frequencies between 4 and 10 Hz, people often experience abdominal discomfort; between 10 and 18 Hz they run to the bathroom more frequently; and between 5 and 7 Hz they experience chest pains.[12]

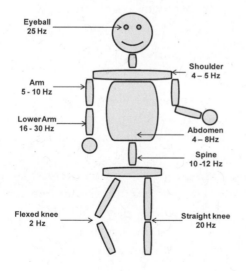

Frequency	Symptoms in the:
4Hz — 5Hz	Digestive system
4Hz — 8Hz	Lungs
4Hz — 10Hz	Abdomen
4Hz — 12Hz	Spinal column
5Hz — 7Hz	Chest
10Hz — 18Hz	Urge to urinate
13Hz — 20Hz	Head
13 Hz — 20 Hz	Vocal cords
12 Hz — 16Hz	Throat

The International Standards Organization recognizes the human body's sensitivity to certain

Dealing with Noise

The Main Concern

The main concern with noise (both audible and inaudible) is that it boosts cortisol levels, provoking alertness during the time we should be sleeping and contributing to the sleep/wake conflict. Figure 3 shows a selection of studies into the sleep and health impact that can have. It only takes a sound five decibels higher than the background level to provoke this conflict. In a very quiet room, that can be as little as a dripping tap. Complaints include sleeplessness, moodiness, fatigue, concentration difficulties, reduced productivity, depression, pain, headaches, dizziness, nausea, pulse irregularities, anxiety, and tinnitus.[13]

Addressing the Concern

Eliminating unwanted sound has been a preoccupation of societies throughout time. Medieval Swedes and Danes absorbed unwanted low frequency sounds by impregnating the walls of their larger buildings with pots. Ancient Greeks and Romans used bronze jars: larger ones to absorb lower frequencies, and smaller jars for higher frequencies. In both cases the open container would trap the sound waves, reducing the energy reverberating through the building. Today we use a similar approach, but substitute open-cell fabrics and materials for the jars.

If you have a noise problem in your bedroom, take a three-pronged approach by absorbing unwanted sounds, reducing the amount of sound entering from outside, and eliminating sources of noise inside.

Absorbing Sound

Porous materials are great at taking the noise energy out of sound waves. Pretty much any open-celled material will trap sound; cotton and wool are ideal. Heavy curtains, towels, fabric wall hangings, pillows, and rugs can all help to reduce room vibrations.

Other porous materials like glass fibre, rock wool, acoustic tiles, and mineral wool can be made into panel absorbers. Stand these absorbers in the corner of the room, since that's where low-frequency sound vibrations tend to congregate. As the sound wave hits the panel, it flexes and vibrates, energizing the trapped air and dissipating it through the absorbent material as heat.

Fig. 3 — The Health Impact of Noise[14]

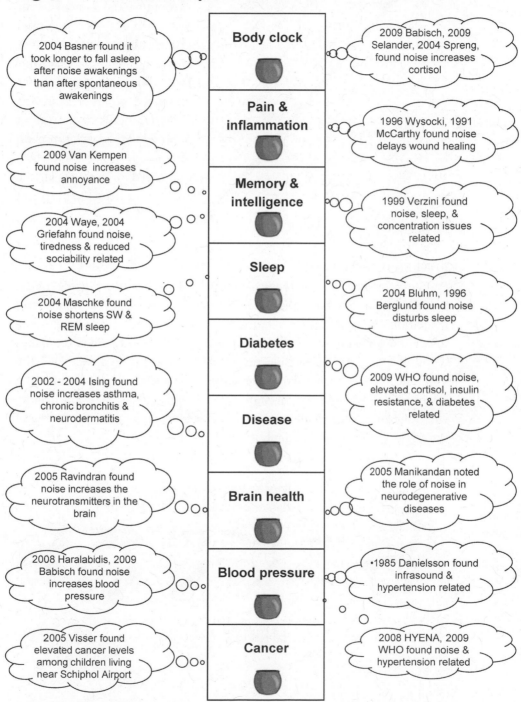

2004 Basner found it took longer to fall asleep after noise awakenings than after spontaneous awakenings

2009 Van Kempen found noise increases annoyance

2004 Waye, 2004 Griefahn found noise, tiredness & reduced sociability related

2004 Maschke found noise shortens SW & REM sleep

2002 - 2004 Ising found noise increases asthma, chronic bronchitis & neurodermatitis

2005 Ravindran found noise increases the neurotransmitters in the brain

2008 Haralabidis, 2009 Babisch found noise increases blood pressure

2005 Visser found elevated cancer levels among children living near Schiphol Airport

Body clock

Pain & inflammation

Memory & intelligence

Sleep

Diabetes

Disease

Brain health

Blood pressure

Cancer

2009 Babisch, 2009 Selander, 2004 Spreng, found noise increases cortisol

1996 Wysocki, 1991 McCarthy found noise delays wound healing

1999 Verzini found noise, sleep, & concentration issues related

2004 Bluhm, 1996 Berglund found noise disturbs sleep

2009 WHO found noise, elevated cortisol, insulin resistance, & diabetes related

2005 Manikandan noted the role of noise in neurodegenerative diseases

•1985 Danielsson found infrasound & hypertension related

2008 HYENA, 2009 WHO found noise & hypertension related

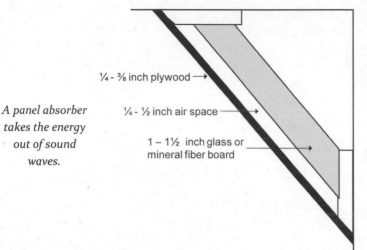

¼ - ⅜ inch plywood →

¼ - ½ inch air space →

1 – 1½ inch glass or
mineral fiber board →

*A panel absorber
takes the energy
out of sound
waves.*

Commercial panel or resonance absorbers are used in recording studios, but it is relatively simple to make your own. The homemade ones illustrated opposite sandwich air space between a layer of plywood and glass or mineral fibreboard. To be effective, they need to have a surface area of at least five square feet.

Preventing Noise Entry

Windows are usually the weakest sound barriers to outside noise. Sometimes that's because they're designed with thermal rather than sound insulation in mind, and sometimes it's because there are gaps in the insulation between the window and the wall. The tiniest hole of 0.1 inches will still allow a 60dB outside noise to be heard inside at 40dB — the difference between a normal conversation level and a whisper. Reinforcing a window as a sound barrier starts with removing the trim and dealing with any gaps in the insulation. Once that's done, replace the trim and seal the edges with a flexible sealant.

*Sound energy is
deflected as the
wave hits each
hard surface.
Placing
absorbent
material
between those
surfaces reduces
vibrations.*

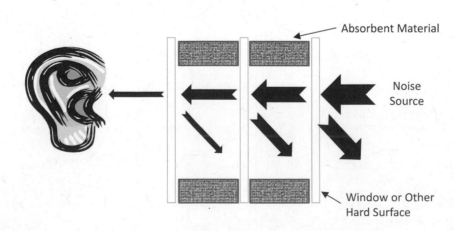

Absorbent Material

Noise
Source

Window or Other
Hard Surface

If the noise remains, the next step is to add a storm window or another layer of glass. A sound-absorbent material added to the inner edges of this additional layer will trap and dissipate any sound energy that gets caught.

If the noise persists you may want to consider floating floors, floating walls, floating ceilings, wall paneling, or even an additional layer of drywall. Depending on where the outdoor sounds are coming from, it may be possible to block them with trees or fences.

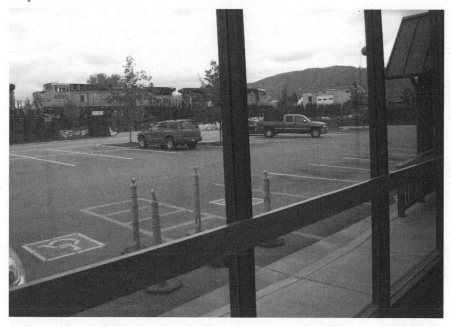

This hotel in Sandpoint, Idaho uses a glass wall and a carpeted floating floor to create a variation on the panel absorber. The train noise is barely audible in the guest rooms.

Photo: *Angela Hobbs*

Eliminating Sources

Noise is often created inside homes by appliances, inadequate maintenance, and ventilation ducts. Many of them don't need to run while we sleep and those that do can often be replaced with quieter alternatives.

Some sounds like dripping taps, rattling pipes, knocking radiators, and chugging toilets can be reduced with basic maintenance.

Some nighttime sounds move through cracks, ventilation ducts, and hollow doors. Fill any cracks or gaps around pipes, doors, and ventilation ducts with a flexible sealant. Hollow doors can be replaced with heavier ones, or can be filled with sand or acoustic tiles. Filling hollow doors with sand gives them the density and mass to be effective noise barriers — just remember to use stronger hinges.

Some gaps under doors, like those that open into apartments from a communal corridor, are part of a positive air-flow system that reduces the risk of fire by keeping up the air pressure in the corridor. Permanently blocking these gaps isn't a good idea, but you can use a temporary draft excluder to reduce sound levels at night.

The troublesome noise from ventilation ducts can be reduced by installing special duct linings, adding bends and air foils, or separating some sections with a decoupling collar. It's important to check with a building inspector to see what's allowed in your area.

Much of the noise in a room can be reduced by preventing the passage of standing waves between hard surfaces. Chairs, tables, bookcases, windows, bed frames, and ventilation ducts often share these vibrations unless a soft surface is sandwiched between them. Cork, rubber and felt pads can all be used to stop vibrations moving between hard surfaces.

Summary

Noise pollution became a real issue during the late twentieth century with the growth of transportation infrastructure, heavy industry, and the entertainment industry. At the same time, new building standards have reduced sound insulation, and new materials and furnishings have removed much-needed vibration diminishers. Increasing numbers of time-saving appliances can easily elevate home noise levels beyond the forty decibels associated with better sleep.

The threat of global warming and diminishing fossil fuel reserves has brought another layer of noise in the form of wind farms. People living in close proximity to wind farms face many of the same health concerns as those living close to busy roads, heavy industry, and airports. But while steps are being taken to address the noise in larger cities, the noise in rural communities remains unheard and unaddressed. Yet both audible and inaudible frequencies elevate cortisol, provoke stress, and stir up a sleep/wake conflict. Both create a level of vibrations in our homes that work against healing therapies based on re-resonating our cells.

Sounds can harm us even when we can't hear them.

4 — Radio Frequency and Micro Waves

Weakening wireless signals that interfere with sleep.

In the last chapter, we saw how noise as a by-product of the entertainment industry and transportation infrastructure gradually evolved into a health concern that cities today are struggling to address. In this chapter, we'll look at the by-product of another infrastructure that promises to evolve into an equally problematic health concern: wireless communication. In the last twenty years, our desire and increasing ability to communicate wirelessly has left us engulfed in the microwaves that carry our comments and commands. Safety concerns about wireless communication have grown right alongside them. Scientists repeatedly confirm that microwaves boost cortisol levels, provoking alertness through the night and contributing to the sleep/wake conflict and many diseases.

In this chapter you'll meet Alice and witness her struggle with microwaves. These are not the microwave ovens that grace our kitchens — those are the least of our worries: we use them for a short time, and most of the beams they create are directed at the food we're heating or cooking. What we're concerned about here are the microwave beams that are aimed at us, day and night. These are the microwave beams emitted by cell towers, airport radars, smart meters, cordless phones, internet routers, and a growing range of wireless devices. We'll look at where these microwaves came from, how different priorities in the East and West influenced their development, how they got into our homes, their use in therapeutic doses, and the impact they have in overdose quantities.

Typically, the word "microwave" refers to a group of artificially produced wavelengths between a millimetre and a metre in length. In this chapter, when I refer to microwaves, I am including radio frequency waves between one and ten metres, as all of these wavelengths raise cortisol levels.

Wavelength	Type	Band	Frequency	Common Uses
1 - 10 mm	Microwave	EHF Extremely High Frequency	30 - 300 GHz	Broadband internet, wireless HD
1 - 10 cm		SHF Super High Frequency	3 - 30 GHz	WLAN, wireless USB, microwave devices, radar
10 - 100 cm		UHF Ultra High Frequency	300 MHz -3 GHz	TV, cell phone, Bluetooth, microwave oven, two-way radio, cordless phone, DECT
1 -10 m	Radio	VHF Very High Frequency	30 - 300 MHz	TV, FM radio, amateur radio, cordless phone, remote control

Alice's Story

By the time Alice called me, she was clearly struggling to keep it together. She was frequently arguing with her adult daughters over silly things — whether to serve rice or potatoes at the family dinner, whether the grandchildren should be in bed by 8 or 8:15, and whether it had rained for one hour or two the day before. The most insignificant things had suddenly become fertile ground for one argument after another.

Alice called me from a hotel she'd booked herself into for the weekend. "I just can't do it anymore; I don't think they want me there anymore," she said. Her palpable desperation made for a very long phone call in which Alice described her situation. She lived with her 17-year-old son and husband of forty years. Her two adult daughters were married; the younger of the two had a son, and the older one had twin daughters. For years she'd been the grandkids' babysitter, enjoying her time at home with them, but now that they were in school, she found herself spending her days in the car picking them up and dropping them off. Some days it was okay, since it guaranteed she'd see her daughters, but some days it was exhausting. It was on one of those exhausting days, four months earlier, that she'd decided to take a trip to visit her family in England. She'd had a joyful reunion with loved ones she hadn't seen in years, she got to meet the newest additions to the family, and she'd returned from her trip refreshed and vibrant, ready to take on the world.

Her homecoming had been exciting with all her children and grandchildren welcoming her at the airport. But with each passing day, she'd sunk deeper into depression until this low point where she'd packed her bag and "run away."

Alice had never struggled with depression before; she'd always slept well and gotten along famously with her husband, children, and grandchildren. Like anyone, she would have the occasional day when her perspective on what was going on around her got a bit "mixed up." She was the first to admit she was no saint, but she'd never experienced anything like the feelings that were overwhelming her now.

Suspecting that her home was somehow involved in her current state of mind, I asked Alice if anything there had changed during her absence. Had anyone brought new equipment into the house — maybe new games that weren't there before she went away? Alice didn't have to think very long. Just before she'd left for England, her son had started a part-time job at the local grocery store. His first goal was to earn enough money to equip the house with a wireless internet router, a cordless phone, and a Wii. Everyone was thrilled because now there was a game to play after the family dinners, they could answer the phone without running to the kitchen, and they could all use their laptops anywhere in the bungalow.

So clearly Alice had come home to a very different house. Everything looked much the same — if a little untidier — but there were things happening in her air that her body wasn't adjusting to. By the end of our call Alice had agreed to call her family and let them know she was okay. She would meet me back at her house the next day.

As Alice led me through her house, she proudly showed me all the new toys her son had bought. The cordless phone sat innocently on her bedside table; the wireless internet router was nicely set up in the office on the other side of the wall — but two feet from the head of her bed. Immediately below her, in the basement, the Wii had been carefully connected to the television. Alice didn't show me the wireless "smart meter" that had been installed by her electricity provider on the outside of her bedroom wall in place of the old mechanical meter that had always measured her electricity.

With four new microwave transmitters all positioned within five feet of Alice's pillow, I knew the readings on my measuring equipment would be high. I hoped that those numbers would help Alice see the disruption provoking her feelings of depression; then she could take action to prevent it from returning. The measuring equipment picked up the four signals loud and clear, and with each transmitter that we unplugged, the signals disappeared. The only remaining strong signal we couldn't remove belonged to the smart meter.

"It feels so much calmer," was all Alice could say when our work was done. "It feels so much calmer." So I left Alice to enjoy the renewed calmness in her air. Over the next few days she would try to get the electricity company to replace the smart meter with a wired meter, and in the meantime she would sleep in one of the other bedrooms.

A week later Alice called again — a much shorter call this time because she was exhausted after all the hustle and bustle of the family dinner. "But this time," she told me, "it's a good exhausted — the familiar kind."

What Alice Did

After her brief experience with microwaves, Alice and her family became far more aware of what was coming into their homes. She decided to enjoy the convenience of the equipment during the day and simply turn it off when the house settled for the night.

Microwave Pollution

Where Did It Come From?

In 1887, when Heinrich Hertz managed to transmit his first radio signal over a few metres, he was ecstatic: he'd found a way to generate and detect radio waves. His work was soon taken to the next level by an enthralled Christian Huelsmeyer, who saw the possibility of using these radio waves to solve the growing problem of ship collisions on the oceans caused by low vision during foggy times. With radio waves, each ship would be able to see its formerly hidden neighbouring vessels, and, while the equipment was bulky and weighty, the ships were big enough to accommodate it.

Sailors loved this new tool that allowed them to "see" into the fog. Before long they were wondering if maybe, with a little tweak, the instrument could tell them more about fog-shrouded ships ahead. With a few adjustments, would they be able to discern the ship's direction, its speed, its size? Yes, it could, but to deliver that level of detail, the instrument would need to produce smaller waves — microwaves — and it would need to produce plenty of them reliably.

By 1935 Henri Gutton had found a way to produce these significantly shorter microwaves. His magnetron was welcomed by ship's crews, who could now not only see into the fog but could also determine how far away the "obstacle" was, whether it was moving, and if so, how fast. But although Gutton's magnetrons were less bulky and smaller than the radio frequency transmitters they replaced, and though they produced the much smaller microwaves, their beams were weak and unreliable. They had that eerie quality of a weak flashlight that can't quite reveal what's lurking in the shadows.

The military was impressed by the sheer level of detailed information that could be communicated by these tiny microwaves. The advantages to equipping military units — whether they were in the air, on land, or at sea — with a microwave tool were obvious. That realization drove efforts to improve the technology's portability and reliability throughout World War II and resulted in several new ways of creating microwaves. By 1943, John Randall and Henry Boot had greatly improved the technology's reliability with their invention of the cavity magnetron, and by 1947, William Shockley had found a way of producing reliable microwaves with very little power. His semiconductor offered all the functions of the magnetron but at a fraction of the cost and size —a quality that opened up a range of commercial opportunities.

By the middle of the twentieth century, a selection of technologies could transmit microwaves through fog, clouds, snow, sleet, walls, floors, and ceilings. While microwaves had started out as a military tool they

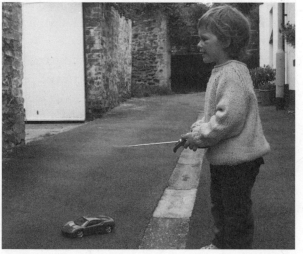

Some of the most entertaining toys and useful equipment exude the microwaves that cause cortisol levels to rise, interfering with quality sleep and all that entails.

Photo:
Nicola Gilbert

transitioned rapidly to being a civilian tool. Transistor radios, televisions, CB radios, microwave ovens and car phones were among the first products to reflect the arrival of microwaves in our daily lives.

Where Did It Go?

The arrival of the semiconductor coincided nicely with postwar challenges. Without the war, the demand for magnetrons dried up, leaving whole skill sets, manufacturers, and microwave experts with nowhere to go. There were only so many microwave ovens to be made — and magnetrons weren't much good for anything else that the public could use. Semiconductors allowed those surplus assets to be put to use in new and different ways. Just how those assets were used depended on whether you were in an Eastern Bloc country or in North America.

In the Eastern Bloc they used the semiconductor to enhance their knowledge of microwave "doses" and "overdoses." As their understanding evolved they developed a range of diagnostic and therapeutic medical equipment, cultivated Microwave Resonance Therapy, and improved their weapons.

Some of these microwave weapons were experienced firsthand by the staff of the American embassy in Moscow during the Cold War. Staff members were so plagued by their symptoms that President Lyndon Johnson eventually asked Prime Minister Kosygin to stop the irradiation that was harming the health of its American citizens. All the fuss and expense that eventually led to the Lilienfeld study,[1] was over a power level between 2 and 28 μW/cm^2 — a level significantly lower than what most North Americans are exposed to today.[2]

Aware of the discomfort microwaves could inflict on people and the health risks associated with all microwave exposure levels, the Eastern Bloc countries exerted great caution about developing products that would increase the exposure of the general public. By exempting the military from the standards set for the general public Russia was able to keep long-term low level exposure to a minimum without threatening the military development of new technologies.[3] This early concern about the health impact of microwave energy dramatically delayed the arrival of microwave ovens, cell phones, and other microwave technologies in the East. Though cell phones and microwaves have become a fixture in today's homes, Russia continues to have the lowest exposure guidelines in the world –

steadfastly refusing to increase them despite the West's persistent requests.

The Dose and the Overdose

Dose — Microwaves as a Therapy

Nikola Tesla and Georges Lakhovsky were instrumental in developing the therapeutic aspect of microwaves — essentially a version of acupuncture that uses microwaves to induce a "healthy" resonance to cells via the meridians. Lakhovsky discovered that the weakened cells could be revived if caught early enough, before pathogens gained entry. Reviving them involved sending a vibration of the right frequency down the meridians to the unhealthy cell, where it would induce the right resonance and restore the cell to health.

Cell state	Cell voltage
Healthy	70 -110 mV
Sick	40 -50 mV
Cancer	20 mV

Resonance therapies like MRT restore the cell's ability to generate the energy it needs to stay healthy.

Initially Tesla and Lakhovsky used a device they called a multiple wave oscillator to generate a range of frequencies from which weakened cells could choose the best alternative. The new semiconductor allowed Sergiy Sitko to take resonance therapy to the next level. Soon Russia and the Ukraine were using microwave therapy effectively to treat ulcers, liver disease, bronchial asthma, bronchitis, diabetes, eczema, addictions, allergies, and immune system disorders.[4] In 1990, Sitko introduced Microwave Resonance Therapy (MRT) to the world at the Annual World Exposition of Innovations, Research and New Technologies in Brussels.

MRT has been slow to gain recognition in North America, but has gradually made inroads into Europe, where its ability to reduce healing time with few side effects was welcomed. Today it is also used in Europe to promote wound healing, stimulate bone marrow stem cell division, reduce the side effects of cancer chemotherapy, and to treat arthritis, ulcers, esophagitis, hypertension, chronic pain, cerebral palsy, and neurological disorders.

Overdose — Microwaves as Health Risk

The West channelled many of its postwar microwave assets into developing therapeutic and diagnostic medical equipment, as well as weapons, but by far the biggest development was in the use of microwaves for communicating over huge distances.

Unlike the differentiated exposure standards set by the Russians, the West set a single standard that would encourage private corporations to develop new technologies. After all, this was a new natural resource that could help governments reach their social and economic goals, as long as they were rapidly made available to everyone. With little of its own research to substantiate the possibility of a harmful effect from exposures that didn't cause heating, the West settled on 'thermal' effects as the bench mark for its standard.

Encouraged by the almost total lack of barriers, entrepreneurs soon found new and ingenious ways to use microwaves and tentacle their wares into the far reaches of society. As long as the products didn't cause irreversible damage to the environment, and as long as they conformed to standards that limited their interference with other products, virtually anything could be brought to the marketplace.

Exposure guidelines for 1800 MHz (cell phones) differ significantly – yet the reception at both power levels is the same

Country	Exposure guideline	A standard that reflects:
ICNIRP		
USA	$1000\ \mu W/cm^2$	little concern for non-thermal effects
Canada		
Russia		
China	$10\ \mu W/cm^2$	significant concern for non-thermal effects
Switzerland		

Cell phones that used these microwaves were quick to catch on and soon enormous base stations, supporting a range of microwave transmitters, were shooting up like angry thistles. No sooner were the towers in place than people began complaining of similar symptoms – often irritability, depression, dizziness and memory issues, if they lived within 100 meters. If they lived a little further away, within 200 meters of the transmitters, they experienced a greater prevalence of headaches, sleep disturbances, and a variety of aches and pains; within 300 meters those symptoms became something of a blur characterized by many as "fatigue".[5]

But cell phone transmitters were far from the only source of microwaves making their way through our walls, floors and ceilings. Soon convenient products that used microwaves in place of electrical wires found their way into our homes and workplaces. The wired internet became wireless, our wired computer and gaming peripherals became wireless, our wired security systems, baby monitors, and doorbells all became wireless, even our corded phones lost their cords as the very microwave overdose conditions that the Eastern Bloc feared materialized in the West.

Soon school boards were installing transmitters in our children's classrooms, utilities were fitting them to our electricity meters, and city transportation staff and community associations were mounting them on lampposts to bring us bus schedules and community internet.

"Don't worry — they're safe" was the phrase echoed in meetings held by city officials and cell phone companies. But safety is a very relative term. According to the Environmental Protection Agency the "safe" or "action" level for radon in a family home (a gas with a broadly recognized health impact) is four picocuries — that's the equivalent health risk of smoking ten cigarettes a day! The "safe" exposure level for something without a broadly recognized health impact is likely to be significantly higher. And beyond Switzerland and Russia, microwaves that don't heat us up, do not have a broadly recognized health impact.

> "That which is looked upon by one generation as the apex of human knowledge is often considered an absurdity by the next, and that which is regarded as a superstition in one century, may form the basis of science for the following one." – **Paracelsus**

Many of our medical professionals and scientists are very concerned that the safety standards set by Safety Code six in 1999 aren't stringent enough to protect us from the multiple microwave sources surrounding us today. If each source has a safety level equivalent to even one cigarette (the current safety level isn't cumulative) then our cradle to grave exposure is likely to result in illness and soaring health care costs — well beyond what any country can manage. These are not exposure sources that should be regulated by people who don't understand the broader implications of their actions.

These same medical professionals and scientists have been watching with horror as our overdose conditions have developed. They know the speeded healing of wounds treated with small microwave doses, and they've treated the stress related illnesses that have increased steadily right alongside the transmitters. But though they've voiced their concerns, they haven't gained much traction.

There seem to be just as many studies confirming the safety of microwaves that don't cause heating as there are studies warning of danger. Typically independent studies reveal effects, while those funded by the wireless industry almost invariably refute it. That strangely even spread may well be related to the way the studies are designed. As long as they're designed to avoid exposing rodents during their sleep — when their cortisol's low and their stress systems are in their recovery phase — the results are likely to be inconclusive or show 'no effect'. Alternatively the studies may be designed like those of chemical corporations' simply using mice that are specially bred not to exhibit the effects that the study's testing for.[6] The data manipulation opportunities seem almost endless.

Dealing with Microwaves

The Main Concern

The main concern with microwaves is that they boost cortisol levels, stimulating the awake system during sleep. This makes them dangerous nighttime guests. Figure 4 shows a selection of studies into the sleep and health impact that can have.

Often people who are concerned about microwaves try to pick out a single specific source — cell phone transmitters, smart meters, wireless internet in school. That's a bit like standing at a busy intersection and deciding that red Hondas are responsible for the traffic noise. We all know that it's the cumulative sound of all the vehicles, and not just the red Hondas, that's responsible. Similarly, we should all realize that it's the cumulative signals of all the microwave sources that are responsible for the overdose we're receiving from wireless devices.

Sources of the microwaves inside homes include cordless phones, wireless routers, Bluetooth devices, kindles, children's wireless toys, remote-controlled lighting, entertainment and security systems, and the wireless peripherals used with computers and gaming consoles. The

Fig. 4 — The Health Impact of Microwaves[7]

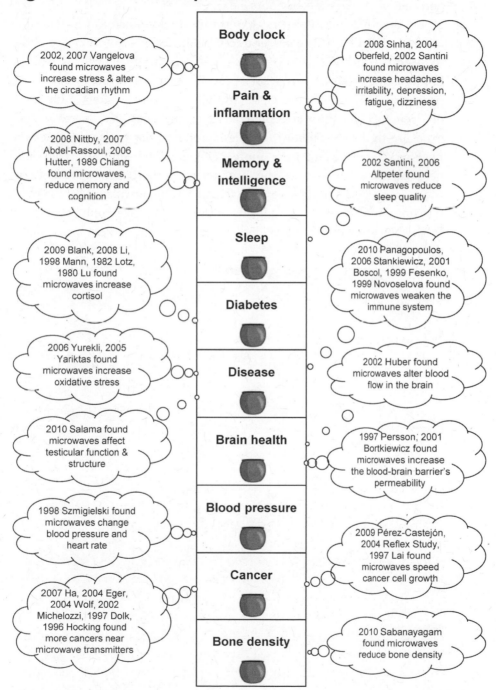

signals from all those transmitters travel unhindered through walls, floors, and ceilings — twenty-four hours a day.

On the whole, city dwellers are more exposed to microwaves than rural folk. City folk usually live nearer to cell phone towers; they may live closer to airports with their strong radar signals; and they may live closer to the broadcasting transmitters that provide their television and radio programs. They usually live closer to their neighbours, often in medium- or even high-density developments. Not only does that increase their exposure to their neighbour's wireless products, but it also increases the likelihood of exposure from more cell phone transmitters. The more people there are in an area, the more potential there is for subscriptions, the more potential profits there are for cell phone providers, and the more transmitters are likely to appear. Although we may only choose to subscribe to one of these providers, we're exposed to radiation from all of them.

Even non-subscriber are exposed to signals. Sometimes there are so many transmitters they have to be represented by a number

Courtesy:
Loxcel.com

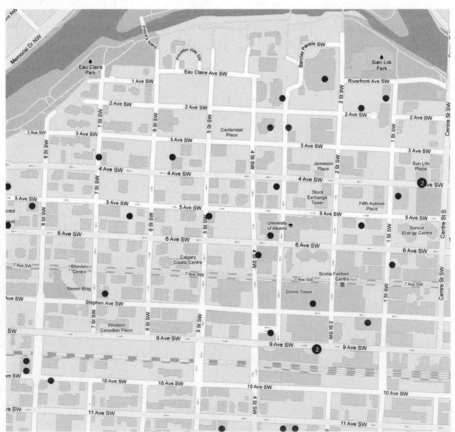

Much of this exposure could be reduced by encouraging cell phone providers to share transmitters, simply by refusing to buy subscriptions if they don't. Not only would that reduce the quantity of transmitters, it would also reduce the copious amounts of energy they're wasting — a single third-generation base station, like the one you pass on the way to work, uses between 430W and 860W, twenty-four hours a day, regardless of how many people are using their cell phones. A recent study estimated that if providers in the United Kingdom shared transmitters it would save 300 GWh per year, that's enough energy to run 70,000 homes, power a third of the London Underground, or even avoid the construction of new power stations.[8]

Addressing the Concern

Preventing microwaves from interfering with your sleep usually boils down to turning off their sources, barricading or weakening them, identifying pillow spots where they're minimal, if not absent, and being aware of the alertness-demanding activities they encourage. Microwaves are probably the most location-specific of all the exposures you'll find in a bedroom. The signals can often be avoided simply by moving sideways by a few inches.

Turning Sources Off

Turning off the wireless gadgets in our homes dramatically reduces microwave levels. Wireless internet routers, cordless phones, baby monitors, Wiis, computer and gaming peripherals, and Bluetooth are all microwave sources that can be turned off at night. They usually aren't being used then anyway.

Cell phones continually send a locator signal to cell transmitters to let them know where they are. The signal on some phones can be deactivated at night by changing the setting to "airplane

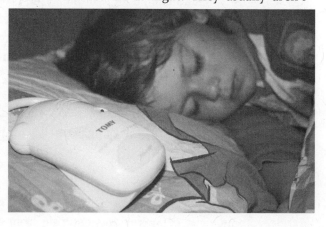

Mom, I'd sleep much better without that transmitter on my pillow!

Photo:
Nicola Gilbert

mode." This setting allows the alarm clock function without the microwaves. If your phone doesn't have an "airplane mode" setting either turn the phone off at night or move it as far from the bed as you can while keeping the alarm in hearing range.

Remote-controlled lighting, security and entertainment systems can be more difficult to turn off at night — it's when it's dark that we want them. Wired systems are safer.

Barricading

Shielding is often used when the source of microwaves is close and very strong, like an airport or military radar that's less than a kilometre away or a cell phone transmitter that's closer than 300 metres. Sometimes shielding can even be used to reduce the strength of the signal coming from a neighbour's wireless equipment. The effectiveness of shielding materials varies considerably, and no one shield blocks everything. Shielding can take the form of wallpapers, foils, fabrics, canopies and paints — a range that allows almost any wall, floor, ceiling or window to be treated.

Shielding materials get their barricading quality from a grounded mesh of conductive carbon, nickel, copper, silver, or steel. As the microwave passes through the material, it's stripped of much of its energy, weakening the beam. That energy is then channeled into the ground where it dissipates as heat. Some of the products are available without grounding, but without the grounding there's nowhere for the energy to go. Since these materials will also trap the electromagnetic fields emitted by household wiring and equipment, you need the grounding to be sure that you don't end up with a more, rather than a less energized room.

Metal shielding, especially if it relies on nickel, copper, or silver for its conductivity, can reduce the air's ion content. Some people who've used canopies and large amounts of these metal-based shielding materials in their bedrooms have found that although the microwave beams are reduced and weakened enough for sleep, their air's ion content is so depleted that it leaves them gagging! (You'll read more about air ions in chapter 8).

Identifying Pillow Spots

After indoor sources have been turned off and shielding is in place to reduce the intensity of microwaves entering from outside, there can still be too many signals hitting the pillow for good sleep. Identifying a good "pillow spot" without the right tools usually means that the sleeper has to test several locations. Initially that may mean reversing the sleeping position so that the head is at the foot of the bed, but it can mean moving the bed a few feet to the left or right. Often the sleeper has to try several different locations around the bedroom, and sometimes in other rooms as well. He usually knows he's found a good spot because he finally falls asleep quickly.

With a tool called a spectrum analyzer, the presence of microwaves (as well as their frequencies and strengths) can be clearly confirmed by placing the antenna on the sleeper's pillow. The antenna can then be moved to other possible pillow locations around the bedroom until it reveals a spot where the beams are absent. These readings have to be taken at night, as daytime and nighttime readings can differ quite dramatically.

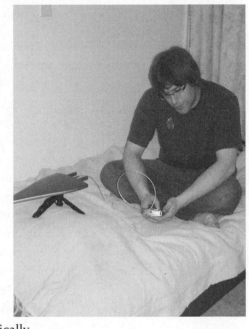

A spectrum analyzer identifies microwaves revealing that Geoff's head isn't the only thing hitting his pillow at night

Photo:
Angela Hobbs

Reducing Alertness-demanding Activities

Traditionally, low light levels in the evening prevented any but the most sedentary activities that made few demands on alertness. These external conditions supported the natural hormone flow: as the need for alertness waned with the light, cortisol dropped and melatonin rose, preparing us for sleep. Microwaves upset that flow, not only because they provoke cortisol, but because they make alertness-demanding activities available to us right up to the last minutes before we drop into bed. Because our cortisol levels still have to fall before we can achieve real sleep, the fall now has to happen during the time that we believe we're sleeping. That means we sleep for less time than we think — which ultimately means we lose out on the sleep cycle at the end of the night that would have made us smart enough to know better!

In today's home, protecting the evening as a time of decompression can be difficult and setting a new pattern can be strenuous. It may take a few weeks to get used to the idea. But turning off the microwaves and toning down evening activities will pay off in longer nights, better-quality sleep, fewer colds, and better grades.

Summary

Microwave technologies really took off with the realization that the tiny waves could transport huge amounts of information. After the Second World War, physicists who'd worked to develop radar had to find new directions for their knowledge. The directions that their knowledge took depended on whether they were in the West, or the East. While the Eastern Bloc concentrated on understanding the health impact of dose and overdose levels, the West concentrated on communication. Those divergent directions ultimately led to today's overdose conditions in the West, compared to a determinedly minimal dose in Eastern Europe.

To enjoy the benefits of wireless communication without the health risks of the overdose, we need to realize that singling out specific exposures as the cause of specific conditions is futile, that overdose solutions lie in an understanding of the cumulative dose, and that turning wireless equipment off at night significantly reduces microwaves' ability to raise our cortisol levels and provoke the sleep/wake conflict.

5 — Light

Darkening the light you think you're used to

Light's ability to disrupt sleep is widely recognized. Almost everyone's familiar with the sleep masks worn by airline passengers, and almost everyone turns off the lights before they settle for the night. But light doesn't just come from the bulbs in our homes; light pollution from street lighting — that we can't just reach out and turn off — has become a significant health concern.

In this chapter, Matt's story illustrates the many sleep problems that light and its inevitable contribution to shift work can have. After Matt's story, we'll look at how Edison's light bulb tentacled its way into every room in every home, putting the power to turn night into day into the flick of a switch. We'll look at how light can be used therapeutically to treat depression and seasonal affective disorder, and at red light's potential to reduce the accidental overdose of light at night.

Matt's Story

For generations, Matt's family had been farmers. But as more and more farms got taken over by large operations, he found it increasingly difficult to make ends meet. With a growing family to support, Matt and his wife decided to sell the family farm and move into the city. He secured a job as a supervisor in a shipping company, working through the night. His wife found daytime work in the local hotel.

They'd been happy for the first year; between them there was enough money coming into the house. The children liked their teachers and easily made friends in their new school. But during the second year, their lives began to unravel. Frequent colds plagued them and threatened their jobs as they took more time off work, either because they themselves were sick or because their children were.

When they did manage to get to work, they found themselves making more and more mistakes. Matt repeatedly missed deadlines and caused customer deliveries to get mixed up; he recorded the wrong weights and ignored some of his employees' most basic safety infringements. Matt knew his employer was receiving complaints; he knew he was being watched. At home, the children's homework and activities seemed to consume every minute. More often than not, they were still looking for their missing shoes as the bell on the school down the street began to chime.

Matt and his wife began to feel that they were playing "catch-up" with every aspect of their lives. They longed for their old life back on the farm. Yes, it had been worrying financially, but somehow the routine had been more manageable when everyone went to bed at night. It was hard to keep the children quiet during Matt's "nights," especially on the days when they were off sick and he was the only adult in the house. Weekends had become a nightmare; the kids resented it when Daddy was in the house, but unavailable.

Matt had clearly gone to some trouble to tidy up his house before he walked me through it. He must have had the impression that I was out to challenge him about the odd speck of dust on his picture frames and the Lego block that hadn't been returned to its box. He was certainly surprised when what I commented on was the lack of curtains and the complete absence of any kind of window covering.

"Have you ever noticed the street light outside your bedroom window?" Matt hadn't. After all, he slept during the day when the street light was off.

"We like the unfettered view when we look out; window coverings always block part of it. Back on the farm we never had curtains, because we had to wake up when the sun rose in the morning — there was always so much that needed doing."

After quite a bit of discussion, Matt understood that there was a good deal more light coming in through his window in the city than there had been on the farm. He was persuaded to cover his bedroom window for his next ten "nights." His wife agreed to keep the coverings up for her next ten nights to block out the street light.

What Matt Did

When I returned to Matt's house two months later, he'd taken a lot less trouble about tidying it up, but every window in the house had heavy curtains; the bedrooms had vertical blinds as well. Life was gradually returning to normal. Matt was making fewer mistakes at work. He didn't feel he was under quite the same degree of scrutiny from his boss and he was getting along with his family. They'd found a few things that they could enjoy doing together during the hours when everyone was awake, and the longing for the old farm days seemed less intense.

Light Pollution

Where Did It Come From?

The developed world has come a long way since the days when 12 hours of darkness was mandatory whether we were asleep or not. Without the means to extend the day artificially, evenings full of concentration-demanding activities were few and far between. You simply couldn't continue daytime activities late into the night, because you couldn't see what you were doing. Although candles and paraffin lamps were commonplace, they were expensive, brought with them a high risk of fire, and had to be carried from room to room. It was far easier for the family to gravitate to one lit room — often the only warm room — than to face the cumbersome reorganization of light sources that would allow more focused tasks.

For most people, dusk signified the end of the work day and its concentration-demanding activities. It signified the start of mellow evenings full of storytelling and conversation, evenings that lasted until exhaustion took hold and everyone curled up and fell asleep. Little did people know how supportive of their natural rhythms these mellow evenings were, in stark contrast to evenings in today's well-lit developed world, where it's not uncommon to find young children on computers, busy with homework or computer games, right up until the moment when they get into bed. Their college-aged siblings are still texting their friends in the early hours of the morning, and their parents are still catching up on emails and work-related activities late into the night. There's nothing mellow about these evenings, and they are not supportive of our natural rhythms and health.

Thomas Edison gets a lot of the credit for enabling our manipulation of the dark and reducing the length of our "rest period" with his electric light bulb. He wasn't the only person developing light bulbs during the 1870s, but unlike his peers, he recognized just how useless light bulbs would be without a distribution system that delivered electricity to them. By offering the world not just a light bulb, but also a system to keep it

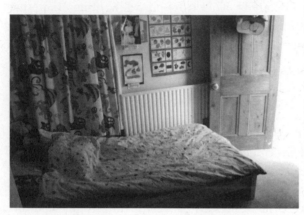

Light can come from every corner of the modern home, rapidly depleting the melatonin responsible for sound sleep and health.

Photo:
Nicola Gilbert

powered, he set himself apart from other inventors. The realization that it wasn't just a bulb that needed to be invented made it possible for Edison to pursue his dream of making "electricity so cheap that only the rich would burn candles."

Where Did It Go?

By the 1880s, electric street lamps were being installed on city streets. Initially welcomed as an amazing innovation, they didn't hold on to their "wow" factor for long. Although crime rates dropped and people felt safer, the lights needed a lot of maintenance and delivered an awfully harsh light. With no question of reverting to dingy unlit streets, the hunt was on for a lower maintenance alternative. High-density discharge lamps seemed to fit the bill.

With an efficient, low-maintenance way of lighting streets leading to an impressive reduction in crime, it didn't take long before all city streets were lit. With time, those same lights would be used to light up yards, parking lots, billboards, and sports facilities. When suburbs began developing around the outskirts of cities, the lights came too.

Today, exterior lighting, whether it comes from our streets, yards, parking lots, billboards, or sports facilities, creates a "sky glow" above some cities that airplane passengers can see from 150 miles. Sky glow has significantly reduced our ability to enjoy the night sky — with all that excess light, many of us can only spot 10 of Orion's 250 stars on a clear, moonless night!

The cost of creating all the light that pours into the night sky, and into our bedrooms, has raised more than a few eyebrows. The International Dark Sky Association estimates that globally, unnecessary nighttime lighting wastes around $1.5 billion per year in electricity. Producing the power necessary to waste all that energy creates about 12 million tons of carbon dioxide and disturbs our sleep too.

The manufacturing industry was the first to exploit the widespread availability of cheap lighting inside. They'd long found it cheaper to leave their machines running through the night than to turn them off and restart them in the morning. But with the availability of cheap electric lighting, manufacturers could turn those unproductive hours into productive ones. There was no shortage of people who were willing to work through the night, and soon the concept of shift work was born. Factories could run early in the day, late into the evening, or through the night; factory owners were delighted to be able to get so much more out of their facilities.

Before long, shift work spread into the hospitality, transportation, and communication sectors. Companies in these sectors saw it as a way of being more available to their customers — of gaining an advantage over their competition. Today about 20 percent of the developed world works through the night.

Inside our homes, light levels rose as desk lamps, ceiling fixtures, and the Light Emitting Diodes on electronic equipment began to grace almost every room. With so many light sources, it became possible to see what you were doing without turning on any lights at all. As more lights appeared in our lives, our body clocks — which depend on light to reset themselves — started receiving conflicting messages.

The Dose and the Overdose

Dose — Light as a Therapy

While artificial light at night reduces melatonin, more light during the day ensures a plentiful supply of it. During daylight melatonin's precursor, serotonin, builds up, reaching higher levels with more daylight. At night all this serotonin gets turned into an ample supply of melatonin.

Light therapy uses this nightly conversion to advantage by increasing the amount of light a person is exposed to during the day. It's often used to treat mood disorders, especially seasonal affective disorder and depression. For people between 15 and 45, depression is the second leading contributor to the global burden of disease.[1] It often affects people with low melatonin levels — those with Alzheimer's, attention-deficit/hyperactivity disorder, anxiety, and substance abuse issues.

The therapy involves using light over 5000 lux at specific times, intensities, and durations, depending on whether the person's melatonin rhythm rises too early or too late in the evening. When it rises too early in the evening, making you drowsy long before bedtime, a bout of bright light in the evening pushes the rise a little later. When it rises too late in the evening, leaving you not the least bit sleepy late into the night, a bout of bright light in the morning can make the rise happen earlier.

The Overdose — Light as a Health Risk

Light overdoses usually result when badly-timed light cues confuse the body's effort to reset its clock. The body gets its light cues from its surroundings through cells in the eye — cells that are far more responsive to blue and white light than they are to red light, moonlight, or starlight. So while a low level of white light can halve our melatonin in 39 minutes,[2] the same amount of red light, starlight, or moonlight has very little impact.

It takes very little of the wrong light to provoke the sleep/wake conflict

Example	Lux
Moonless clear night	0.002
Full moon (clear night)	0.27
One candle	1
Family living room	50
Office lighting	320 - 500
Full daylight	10,000 - 25,000
Direct sunlight	32,000 - 130,000

Studies into the health impact of excessive nighttime lighting have focused on three groups of people: the visually impaired, shift workers, and transatlantic travelers.

The visually impaired provide an interesting comparison group because many of them don't receive the light cues that the visually acute population receives. Without this melatonin depleter, they are far less prone to cancers of the breast, prostate, stomach, colon, rectum, skin, and lungs.[3]

Shift workers who work through the night have to flip their sleep and awake systems: their sleep system works during their (artificial) night, and their awake system goes to work during their (artificial) day. But there's a limit to how many time cues they can block out — there are always reminders that others are awake and that it's not really night.

A healthy shift-working life is probably only possible for a single person living in a detached home on a huge rural acreage with friends that share the same shift. For anyone else, especially those experiencing ever-changing combinations of late night and early morning shifts (think health care, airlines, and emergency services) the constantly changing light cues keep their body clocks in a state of limbo. Many shift workers add to that limbo by eliminating evenings from their routine. Without this wind-down time that supports cortisol's fall and melatonin's rise, part of their night is lost. Without this awake-to-sleep transition period, they tend to lose out on part or all of their stage 5 REM sleep at the end of the night. This limbo has such a dire impact on the body clock that the World Health Organization recognizes shift work as a probable human carcinogen.[4]

Transatlantic travellers experience what is probably the most extreme symptom of body-clock limbo — jet lag. Jet lag is usually worst for people travelling east, especially if they cross multiple time zones. For some people, going to bed earlier for a couple of nights helps their body clocks reset, but for others the expectation of dinner at breakfast time, the alertness peak at bedtime, the headaches, exhaustion, irritability, depression, sleep problems, and food indigestibility can persist for weeks.

Some scientists are concerned that the body-clock limbo induced by jet lag should be taken more seriously. One study

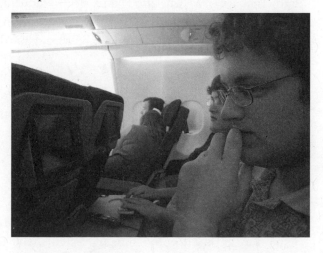

Light from entertainment systems at head height do little to give airline passengers a head start on their inevitable phase shift.

Photo: *Angela Hobbs*

showed a 50 percent death rate in mice after a six-hour eastward phase shift.[5]

Dealing with Light

The Main Concern
The main concern with light is that it depletes melatonin levels, provoking the sleep/wake conflict. Figure 5 shows a selection of studies into the sleep and health impact that can have. Without adequate levels of melatonin, we're more likely to wake up and start doing things that increase our alertness further. Every time we indulge wakefulness during our sleeping time, we increase our body-clock limbo. That indulgence may take the form of turning on a light to read, checking phone messages, getting up to make sure the kids are covered, or any other activity that increases our state of alertness. Without its proper nightly rhythm, melatonin can't coordinate the many bodily functions we rely on for sleep and health.

Addressing the Concern
Light gets into bedrooms from both outside and inside our homes. Outdoor sources include street lights, billboards, sports fields, and traffic. Common indoor sources include the LED displays of radio alarms and night lights. Since melatonin levels drop by 50 percent after only 39 minutes of exposure to a 40-watt light bulb, pretty much any unnatural light that isn't red will affect your sleep. Reducing light in the bedroom usually involves barricading it from entry, turning off lights inside, and replacing those that need to remain on through the night with red lights.

Barricading
About 60 percent of the world's population is subjected to the kind of excessive lighting that lets you see shadows and pick out furniture when the lights are off. Unless it's a moonlit night, neither should be possible. If you are able to see shadows or pick out the furniture block out more of the outside light with heavy curtains.

Turning Inside Lights Off
Much of the light in bedrooms comes from inside the home — the hall light, the LEDs on entertainment systems, the fish tank. Almost all of

Figure 5 — The Health Impact of Light[6]

| Body clock | |
| 2003 Blask, 2001 Whitmore, 1996 Trinder found constant light suppresses melatonin | 2005 Duffy, 2005 Cajochen, 2001 Thapan, 2001 Brainard found melatonin most sensitive to blue light |

Body clock

Memory & intelligence

Sleep

Diabetes

Disease

Brain health

Blood pressure

Cancer

Bone density

2003 Blask, 2001 Whitmore, 1996 Trinder found constant light suppresses melatonin

2005 Duffy, 2005 Cajochen, 2001 Thapan, 2001 Brainard found melatonin most sensitive to blue light

2008 Haines found 70% of shift worker's psychological symptoms are shift-related

2009 Lewy noted mood disturbances and delayed melatonin related

2007 Pandi-Perumal, 2001 Lavie found the melatonin rise initiates sleep

1994 Tokura found bright light by day enhances sleep at night

2006 Davidson found a six-hour eastward phase shift killed half his mice

2006 Suwazono found diabetes significantly higher in shift workers

2010 Kyriacou found disrupting the body clock impacts mental health

2005 Ishida found cortisol rises in response to blue light

1989 Kristensen, 1999 Knutsson found heart disease significantly higher in shift workers

2010 Ben-Shlomo, 2008 Kloog 2006 Stevens, 2005 Blask, 2001 Hansen found lighting and breast cancer related.

2006 Pukkala found less prostate & breast cancer in the visually impaired

2003 Ostrowska found light and bone metabolism related

2008 Srinivasan noted the melatonin surge restrains tumour growth

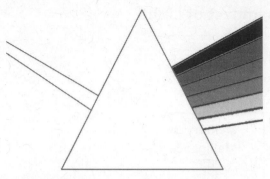

White light is made up of a rainbow of colours, each with a different wavelength. Red light is far less disruptive than either blue or green

these lights can be turned off for the night. In some cases that may mean unplugging the equipment from the wall socket, covering it, or turning it towards the wall. For new gadgets choose the alternative with red lights.

Replacing

When lights need to be left on through the night, replace the bulbs with red lights. Since reptiles share our sensitivity to white light these red light bulbs can often be found in pet stores.

It's not unusual to reach the point of "If I don't go to bed right now, I'll be sleeping right here!" at the end of the day, only to find that you're wide awake after ablutions in bright light. Installing a lower-wattage light in the bathroom, may help. But if it doesn't then return to the spot where you were falling asleep (your body's identified it as safe). Sleep there until you've fixed your bedroom.

Summary

Since Edison's first public demonstration of the incandescent light bulb at Menlo Park in 1879, artificial light has become omnipresent. It offers several advantages to industry, businesses, and homes, but like all the waves of the electromagnetic spectrum, it takes as much as it gives if we don't handle it with care. The right, well-timed light dose can do wonders for depression and seasonal affective disorder, but the wrong, poorly-timed light dose disrupts our hormones and provokes a sleep/wake conflict. When that disruption becomes habitual, it can contribute to a variety of diseases and conditions.

Usually, the most difficult part is recognizing that light is a problem in the first place. Often people get used to sleeping with light and assume it isn't doing any harm, but just because it doesn't wake you up fully doesn't mean it isn't reducing your melatonin below the levels needed for health.

6 — Household Electricity & the Earth's Magnetic Fields

Draining the energy intruding on your sleep

Most of us are surrounded by gadgets and appliances powered either by electricity or a battery. Simply settling down to watch your favourite television program, you may be surrounded by electricity in the form of the TV, DVD and PVR, a light, the base station for your phone, a surge protector, and an electric clock. Even once you're in bed, you may still be affected by many of those gadgets and appliances. They may not be in the same room, but that doesn't matter, because the electromagnetic fields (EMFs) they produce travel straight through walls, floors, and ceilings. In most cases, that means that you're also affected by the fridge, dishwasher, and CD player in the kitchen, the electric panel below you in the basement, and the electric toothbrush and shaver recharging through transformers in your bathroom.

In this chapter, we'll look at how layers of electromagnetic fields are created by the flow of electricity to the electrical equipment around us, and how they build up and affect our sleep and health. We'll start by looking at how those many layers devastated little Stefan's life after he moved into an apartment building. Then we'll go on to look at where these many layers came from and how they became so prevalent in our homes. We'll begin with the layer that's naturally produced by the earth, and then go on to look at the electricity used in our homes (at 50 Hz in Europe and 60 Hz in North America). All of these are known as Extremely Low Frequency (ELF) waves. These long waves have the strong penetration characteristics that make them useful for communicating with submerged submarines over great distances — a characteristic that makes them difficult to contain once they've been created, and one that allows them to travel unhindered through our walls, floors, and ceilings.

Stefan's Story

Stefan, a ten-year-old boy with curly blond hair and hauntingly vacant eyes, met me at the door of the apartment he shared with his mother and sister. He showed me into the living room, where his mother was waiting to meet me.

Stefan's teachers were recommending Ritalin, but his family doctor, who had watched his development since birth, had insisted that Stefan's mom talk to me before he would consider prescribing it. He felt that there had to be something else behind the sudden change in this little boy, who had recently turned from a cooperative, smart, loving child into an aggressive youngster with poor grades and behavioural problems.

A portion of the change in Stefan could be attributed to his parents' recent divorce and the move out of his family home. The change had certainly started within a couple of weeks of the move, but initially his mother had thought he just needed time to adjust. Six months later, his "time" was up. His teachers were complaining about him; his grades had dropped; he was surly, distractible, and aggressive; and he had lost all interest in his friends.

I wasn't surprised that he hadn't wanted to sit with us — after all, he was going to be discussed — but I was surprised when, instead of going into his own room, he went into his sister's room. Mom must have registered my surprise, because she quickly explained that "he only uses his room for sleeping because it makes him feel sick." Her comment summed up her total lack of recognition of the impact an environment can have on a person — and that meant it would be challenging to make any real headway.

Stefan's mom had already tried to modify his behaviour with dietary restrictions, but that had been a total failure, which had left her extremely skeptical of any environmental explanations. She felt that he would just have to get over his "room rejection." She was tired of fighting with her child, tired of the complaints about him, and tired of the guilt she felt over the divorce. For her, relief would come in the little pill that she wanted the doctor to prescribe her son; agreeing to see me was just part of her strategy for getting it.

The visitors' parking area outside the apartment building faced a row of twelve electric meters. I'd cringed as I'd pulled up, hoping that Stefan's room was on the other side of the building, but as his mother showed me into his room, my biggest fear for the child was confirmed. His neatly made metal-framed bed, complete with a cozy star-studded polyester comforter, was right up against that same wall. That meant that, every night, all the electricity that fed the eight apartments in

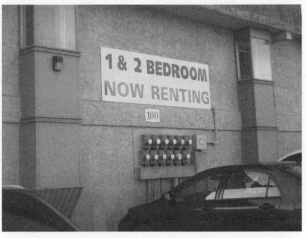

Positioning beds anywhere near the electricity's entry into a home ensures that the sleep/wake conflict will be provoked

Photo: *Angela Hobbs*

the complex streamed within a foot of Stefan's head. That said, it was a nice, big room — big enough for a comfy computer nook, complete with a surge protector. There was still plenty of space to stand all the boxes that had moved with them out of their former home. To help deal with all the dust and dander left by the previous tenants, his mom had put in an air purifier, but she wasn't sure it was doing much because even after running it flat-out, the air in the room still seemed "thick" to her.

Every corner of the apartment bore witness to the time, energy, and effort Stefan's mom was making to create a welcoming and wholesome new home for her children. The apartment was small but clean, tidy, and comfortable — not at all a home where kids would be nervous about bringing their friends. But seen from the perspective of confusing the sleep and awake systems, it told a very different story.

I could well understand that Stefan's room made him feel sick. No one would have been able to sleep well in there. Not only was there a huge source of EMFs from all the power passing through the electric meters on the outside wall, but Stefan's metal bed frame could amplify them. The synthetic fabrics of his bedding and sleepwear would hold any charge right next to his skin. The air purifier, computer, and surge protector would be adding their own EMF exposures to this toxic brew.

With mom just wanting to tell the doctor that I'd been, Stefan's best chance of recovery lay in persuading his mother to move him out of his bedroom. So I handed her my Gauss meter (a device that measures magnetic fields), and sent her on a walk through the apartment. She started in her bedroom, and was stunned to see it was "reading" something invisible in the air. Then she slowly made her way down the corridor, passed her daughter's room, passed the living room, and passed the kitchen, watching the meter's numbers rise with each step.

"What happened?" she asked. I knew she had just seen the numbers on the meter increase dramatically. "What is this?" A very dismayed mom had just discovered the invisible, but very real, difference between her bedroom and her son's.

"Those are the magnetic fields that are interfering with your son's sleep," I answered.

It took several walks down the corridor before she was sure that the meter wasn't faulty, but by the end of the evening she was convinced enough to move Stefan's bed into his sister's room, much to the little girl's disgust.

Two weeks later, Mom had her little boy back. With some sense of normalcy restored, the siblings had discovered some of the joys of room sharing; talking themselves to sleep had become the highlight of their time together. Now when Mom settled her children for the night, she could sit back with her cup of tea, turn down the volume on the television, and listen to the gentle, contented chatter from the children's bedroom. No longer did she sit listening for the thud of Stefan hitting the floor as he fell out of bed, a thud that had invariably come within half an hour of putting him to bed. No longer did he disturb her nightly peace with his endless complaints of "feeling sick."

What Stefan's Mom Did

Simply distancing Stefan from the source of all that power by moving him out of out of his bedroom reduced many of the electromagnetic fields around him. Most nights he shared his sister's bedroom, but on the occasional night when they weren't getting along, he would sleep in the living room. Stefan's old bedroom became a storage room and his computer found a new niche in the corner of the living room. At bedtime, Stefan's mom unplugged the surge protector and computer.

Electromagnetic Pollution

Where Did It Come From?

North Americans, and some Europeans, tend to be a bit skeptical about the impact electromagnetic fields can have on our sleep, health, and behaviour. But the recognition of that impact has a long history that dates right back to the Stone Age. These early peoples were keenly aware of the earth's powers — powers created by the movement of the Earth's molten core and distorted by streams; geological fault lines; rock fissures; mineral seams; and coal, oil, and iron deposits. These distortions of the earth's magnetic field, that were usually stronger during the spring and summer, left obvious marks on the unadulterated landscape. They were often patches where grass refused to grow, where lightning struck frequently, where trees grew twisted and were plagued with bulbous tumours, and where certain insects were more inclined to make their homes.

With their strong belief in the spirit world, many early peoples came to associate these odd patches of land with special powers. Many envisioned them as the places where an invisible world tree provided their ancestors with a thoroughfare between the "underworld," the "middle world," and the "upper world." [1]

Over time, elaborate histories of place became attached to these locations. The Celtic traditions had their fairy paths, the Chinese had their feng shui teachings, and the Indians had their vastu shastra traditions. All of these traditions, and many more in other cultures, warned of the dangers that came with building homes that interfered with the earth's energies; these became sacred sites that reflected reverence...and warning.

That reverence for sacred sites, the folklore that accompanied them, and the tendency of new religions to speed conversion by building their churches on them, protected communities from the Earth's magnetic fields. People simply wouldn't build their homes in places where there was a revered monument, or stories warning of danger. Until recently the notion of converting churches into dwellings was an absurdity.

But as communities expanded onto undeveloped land, settled new lands, and sprang up in new areas in response to growing demands for coal, iron, oil, gas, and other mineral deposits, it became more costly and more difficult to pay attention to sacred sites that hadn't been recognized with monuments. If there were enough monuments to serve the needs of

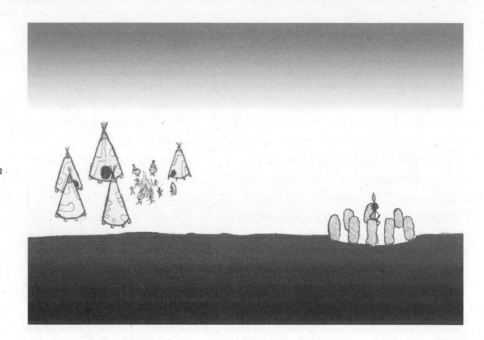

To the uninitiated a Native American summer scene might look like this...

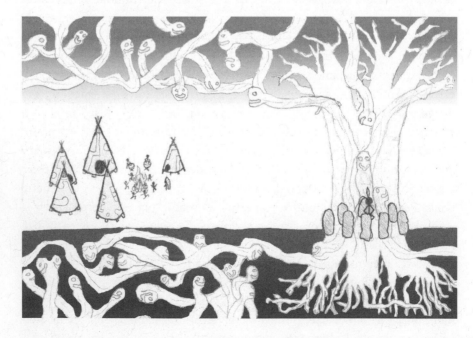

...but it might look like this to someone with an animistic world view. They would recognize the ethereal world 'tree' allowing ancestral spirits to move between worlds offering guidance with each encounter,

***Illustrations:**
"The World Tree"
by Chris Hobbs*

the people, remaining sacred sites could be ignored and the land used for housing — at least in some cultures. The concerns of people who'd witnessed the impact of the Earth's powers were dismissed and adherents were discredited as naysayers who stood in the way of progress. But although the recognition of the earth's magnetic fields faded, their powerful health impact remained.

While the Inuit, Chinese, and Indian cultures evolved with a strong "history of place" that embodied a respect for the Earth's energies, much of Europe and North America underwent a shift toward a "history of chronological dates" that required an almost systematic dismissal of folklore. This left them extremely vulnerable to the health impacts of the Earth's powers, and may well be a contributing factor to the high rates of multiple sclerosis in communities built in areas where the Earth's magnetic fields are badly distorted.[2]

Among the most dramatic examples of this vulnerability is the high incidence of multiple sclerosis in Black Diamond and Turner Valley. These towns nestled in the foothills of the Rocky Mountains in Alberta, Canada appeared suddenly during the twentieth century following the discovery of oil. The terrain, with all its fissures, mineral deposits and underground streams, was valuable to settlers and those who wished to exploit its resources; they paid little attention to the native population's warnings about the area's strong energies. The gradual conversion to Christianity that took place elsewhere never happened, sacred sites never evolved into churches, leaving the land free for residential development and the population exposed. Today, Turner Valley and Black Diamond have the highest rates of multiple sclerosis in the world, while MS rates among Alberta's First Nations, 70 percent of whom live on reservations on less valuable land nearby, are significantly lower.[3]

Several communities that grew

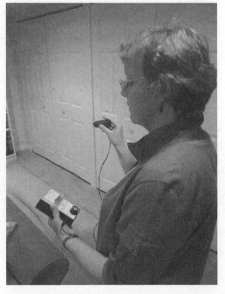

A DC magnetic field meter detects distortions in the earth's magnetic field in this Calgary home

***Photo:**
Angela Hobbs*

up on land with similar characteristics to Black Diamond and Turner Valley also have high rates of multiple sclerosis. Among them are communities that developed in Yorkshire and southern Scotland during the Industrial Revolution in response to growing demands for coal. Other communities include many of those in Ireland's Donegal County; Scotland's southeast and Shetland and Orkney Islands; northern Sweden; and southeastern Norway. In some cases, the mineral deposits that attracted the people to these areas were even identified using the very distortions in the Earth's magnetic fields that may be contributing to their health issues.

Communities built in areas where the earth's magnetic fields are distorted by mineral deposits, fault lines, rock fissures, and underground streams have significantly higher rates of multiple sclerosis.

Country	Place[4]	M.S. Rate (per 100,000 people)
Global	**Global Median**	30
USA	National Median	135
Canada	National Median	132
Canada (Alberta)	Black Diamond & Turner Valley	354
	First Nations	100
Sweden	Västerbotten	170
	Norrbotten	253
Northern Ireland	Donegal	168
United Kingdom	Southeast Scotland	187
	Orkney Islands	193
	Shetland Islands	152
Finland	Seinäjoki	211
Norway	Southeast	188
China	National Median	2

Where Did It Go?

During the early twentieth century, the impacts of Earth's magnetic field on health were regaining recognition in parts of Europe — just in time to witness an explosive growth in appliances and gadgets that worked using this same ELF portion of the electromagnetic spectrum, and a growing demand for more power.

Early electricity distribution was primarily aimed at providing enough power for incandescent lights. Direct current (DC) at a very low voltage was created in local generators within a couple of kilometres of the customer. From here, it travelled efficiently down thick, heavy cables to the light bulb.

As more electrically-operated products were invented, demand for electricity naturally increased, and it became apparent that the DC distribution system was too cumbersome and expensive to accomodate the demand. The thick cables that worked so well over short distances and for low demand were simply too heavy to carry more power to larger areas. Two solutions were offered, one by Thomas Edison, the other by George Westinghouse.

Thomas Edison believed the best solution was to continue the use of direct current (DC power) with each household having large "batteries" in the garden shed to power its own needs. He showcased his design in his own home in Llewellyn Park, New Jersey. The three-part battery containing oil, water, and gasoline could power everything from his lights to his toothbrush sanitizer and foot warmer for about three days. After three days the discharged battery was recharged while the house slept. Initially Edison used a gasoline generator to recharge the system, but he planned to replace it with wind power. His system would inhale wind and exhale electricity.

George Westinghouse believed the solution was to use high-voltage alternating current (AC power) to drive electricity from power stations to local substations. Once the electricity reached the local substation, it would be transformed to lower voltages and delivered to homes. The higher voltages and alternating current could use thinner wires without losing large amounts of electricity along the way. Using thinner, lighter wires meant electricity could make longer journeys and that, in turn, meant that the power stations could be located further from the cities, in areas where the coal used to fuel them was abundant.

Around the same time as Edison and Westinghouse were duking out the question of the delivery system, early car manufacturers were exploiting every opportunity to persuade the public that faster, noisier gasoline-powered cars were more "manly" and adventurous than their quiet, sissy battery-powered counterparts. This campaign contributed to the ultimate rise of the AC system and the demise of the DC system.

For a long time the only real problem with the AC distribution system, at least where residences are concerned, lay in the strong electromagnetic fields that radiated out from the power lines and substations onto the land below and around them. In some cities, that land was restricted to non-residential use — golf courses, churches, shopping malls, and playing fields — but in others, it was sold cheaply to developers. Land developers knew it was worth their while building on the cheap land; there would always be unsuspecting buyers looking for a good deal. Often an extra garage, a classier finish, an additional room, or a yard that was just a little bigger than the one next door would seal the deal.

With the AC system reliably distributing power over long distances, our electrical appliances and gadgets multiplied. However, much of the new equipment — laptops, shavers, radio alarms, electric toothbrushes — uses DC power. In order to work, the new equipment needs a battery or a transformer that converts AC to DC power.

So now we are subjected not only to the first layer of electromagnetic fields from power lines, substations, and wires in the walls of our homes, not only to the second layer created by the electrical appliances that used the power, but also to a third layer created by the transformers that turn electricity from its AC state into DC. Everything that has a "battery power" configuration, from laptops and radios to electric clocks and music systems, comes with a transformer built either into the unit or into its plug. If your house is located in an area where the earth's magnetic fields are strong, there's even that fourth natural layer to contend with. For those who've opted for solar or wind energy to supplement their electrical needs, there's a fifth layer. This equipment creates DC power that can be used right away, stored in a battery for later use, or sold to the electricity grid. Before it can be used or sold, this power has to be converted to the AC power of those systems. This conversion is done by an inverter — a piece of equipment that creates strong electromagnetic fields as it works.

Together, all these layers cause untold disruption to our sleep and health.

The Dose and the Overdose

The Dose — Electromagnetic Fields as a Therapy

Although North America and much of Europe have been almost systematically dismissive of the health impact that distortions in the earth's magnetic field can have, there have been some developments in healing techniques that use those same frequencies (between 5 and 20 Hz). In 1997, Gary Hasey opened the first North American clinic to offer transcranial magnetic stimulation in Canada. The therapy uses short bursts of magnetic fields to disrupt nerve cell activity and melatonin concentrations. Depending on the frequency and the area of the brain that's targeted, the therapy can either increase or decrease the activity of the nerve cells. It has been used successfully to treat mood disorders, anxiety, depression, Parkinson's, multiple sclerosis, and migraine.[5]

The medical use of electromagnetic fields in the higher "household electricity" range is well developed. EMFs are recognized for their ability to dilate blood vessels, thereby affecting breathing, heart rate, and blood pressure. It is medically accepted that extremely weak fields administered at the right frequency and location can be used to promote the healing of complicated bone fractures; relieve pain, depression, anxiety, and insomnia; treat seizures and osteoarthritis; accelerate the healing of soft tissue wounds; and support the immune system by increasing the presence of natural killer cells.

Some of the more popular therapies include:

Electroacupuncture

Electroacupuncture is used to enhance or replace the manual needling used in acupuncture. The resonances travel down the meridians stimulating appropriate resonances in sick cells. It's widely used to relieve pain and has also been used to alleviate the side effects of chemotherapy, induce delivery in post-term pregnancies, and treat renal colic.

Transcutaneous Electrical Nerve Stimulation (TENS)

TENS is used by physiotherapists to relieve pain. Various stimulators are used to stimulate the nerves below their excitation threshold in the areas that hurt.

Transcranial Electrostimulation (TCES)

TCES is used to modify behaviours by stimulating nerves in the brain. Like TENS, it uses stimulation levels below the nerve's excitation threshold.

Neuromagnetic Stimulation

This therapy is can be used in place of electroshock therapy in treating major depression, seizures, and even carpel tunnel syndrome.

The Overdose — Electromagnetic Fields as a Health Risk

In parts of Europe, the health impact of too much exposure to the earth's magnetic field became increasingly recognized throughout the twentieth century. Baron von Pohl, a doctor who worked with cancer patients, noticed that they slept in areas where the magnetic fields were strong. He discussed his research and patients in his 1932 book *Earth's Currents*.[6] Dr. Ernst Hartmann, who would go on to found a centre dedicated to researching the health impacts of environmental interactions, the Forschungskreis Fuer Geobiologie, published his book *Illnesses as a Problem of Location* after finding that patients sleeping over magnetic fields suffered from weakened immune systems.[7] Hans Nieper, too, drew attention to the recurrent symptoms of his patients sleeping over strong magnetic fields when he published his book *Revolution in Technology, Medicine and Society* in 1985.

In the late twentieth century, some research began to reveal a relationship between leukemia and the electricity carried into homes on wires. Nancy Wertheimer and Ed Leeper's[8] research into the connection was soon corroborated by studies in Sweden,[9] Germany,[10] and America. An American study in 2001 compared electrified and non-electrified populations between 1920 and 1960; the results so alarmed

The profusion of electrical equipment in a child's bedroom pushes the electromagnetic fields up into the 2-4 milligauss range associated with leukemia

Photo:
Nicola Gilbert

researchers Samuel Milham and Eric Ossiander that they asserted:

"75 percent of childhood acute lymphoblastic leukemia and 60 percent of all childhood leukemia may be preventable."[11]

In today's homes, layer after layer of electromagnetic fields can build up very quickly, even in homes not located under power lines. Electricity-carrying wires, of course, are built right into the walls and floors of every home in North America. The electricity flowing to and fro in those wires creates electromagnetic fields before we ever plug our appliances and gadgets into the outlets. Those wires are located at almost perfect head height for a person lying down on a bed. Outlets are often positioned at just that height, increasing the likelihood that EMF-generating gadgets will be plugged into them all night long. Recharging the cell phone is often the last thing people think of as they get into bed, and typically if there isn't a recharging mat then there's a whole range of recharging bases, complete with transformers, neatly arranged on the bedside table — one for the iPod, another for the shaver, one for the cell phone or BlackBerry.

In many houses, there's a plentiful supply of wires running under beds, too, which can be a concern if the appliances they serve use power during the night. This can be more of a concern for little children who go to bed while the house is still active. Sometimes they spend several hours in a bed above a fluorescent light in the ceiling of the bathroom below their bedroom. Their beds may share a wall with the kitchen or laundry area, putting their little heads just inches from appliances like fridges, freezers, stoves, and dryers that use a lot of electricity and create large electromagnetic fields.

As new materials have entered the market, the conductive materials that used to carry electromagnetic fields to ground have been replaced

Appliance	mG at 12" (approx)
Dishwasher	100
Washing machine	100
Electric clock	60
Microwave oven	60
Battery charger	20
Analog battery clock	15
Electric range	20
Television	10
Fluorescent light	10
Fax machine	10
Clock radio	5

Many appliances have strong magnetic fields. These drop rapidly with distance, becoming almost negligible at around two metres

with materials that don't — for example, the pipes of sewage and water systems that used to be metal are now usually plastic. The absence of these grounded systems leaves many more electromagnetic fields in the living area. These can end up in the ungrounded metal of wall framing, metal beds and the coils of spring mattresses where they can create a standing wave and radiate electromagnetic fields.

Space-saving furniture can make the most efficient use of a child's small bedroom. This furniture usually looks like a bunk bed with a table replacing the lower bunk. Usually the table is used as a desk, seemingly the perfect location for a computer and printer. However, configuring the room like this means that these strong electromagnetic fields are right below your sleeping child, night after night.

Space-saving furniture in small bedrooms leaves plenty of space for more stuff. This often takes the form of more gadgets and a surge protector to keep the stuff safe! Unfortunately, the more numerous the sources of electromagnetic fields, the stronger their cumulative effect. It doesn't matter whether the gadgets receive their power from an electrical outlet or from a battery. If they receive power, they create EMFs, and some of the strongest fields among gadgets are created by battery-driven clocks with clock faces and moving arms.

Dealing with Electromagnetic Fields

The Main Concern

The main concern with electricity and magnetic fields is that they deplete melatonin. Figure 6 shows a selection of studies into the sleep and health impact that can have. Electromagnetic fields aren't deterred by walls, floors, or ceilings, and that gives them a level of influence over our sleep and health that most of the other bedroom conditions don't have. Unlike light, they can't be blocked by heavy curtains, and unlike chemicals, they can't be reduced by simply closing the bathroom door.

The EMFs that penetrate our bedrooms may come from the wires distributing electricity through the neighbourhood and through our homes. They may come from the appliances, magnetic recharging mats, compact fluorescent light bulbs and gadgets we've plugged into the outlets, they may come from the transformers that convert alternating

Fig. 6 —The Health Impact of EMF's[12]

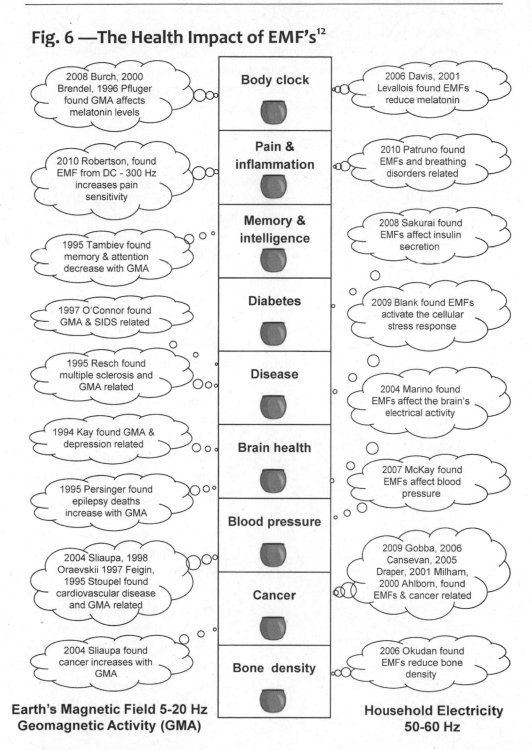

2008 Burch, 2000 Brendel, 1996 Pfluger found GMA affects melatonin levels

2006 Davis, 2001 Levallois found EMFs reduce melatonin

Body clock

2010 Robertson, found EMF from DC - 300 Hz increases pain sensitivity

2010 Patruno found EMFs and breathing disorders related

Pain & inflammation

1995 Tambiev found memory & attention decrease with GMA

2008 Sakurai found EMFs affect insulin secretion

Memory & intelligence

1997 O'Connor found GMA & SIDS related

2009 Blank found EMFs activate the cellular stress response

Diabetes

1995 Resch found multiple sclerosis and GMA related

2004 Marino found EMFs affect the brain's electrical activity

Disease

1994 Kay found GMA & depression related

Brain health

1995 Persinger found epilepsy deaths increase with GMA

2007 McKay found EMFs affect blood pressure

Blood pressure

2004 Sliaupa, 1998 Oraevskii 1997 Feigin, 1995 Stoupel found cardiovascular disease and GMA related

2009 Gobba, 2006 Cansevan, 2005 Draper, 2001 Milham, 2000 Ahlbom, found EMFs & cancer related

Cancer

2004 Sliaupa found cancer increases with GMA

2006 Okudan found EMFs reduce bone density

Bone density

Earth's Magnetic Field 5-20 Hz Geomagnetic Activity (GMA)

Household Electricity 50-60 Hz

current to direct current, they may come from faulty wiring and dirty grounding, and they may come from the earth. As each of those layers builds up around the bed, the area gets ever closer to reaching the 2-4 milligauss associated with reduced, ineffective melatonin, poor sleep, ill health, and an increased risk of childhood leukemia.

Addressing the Concern

Consider adopting practices like turning off circuits at night, unplugging appliances and gadgets when they aren't in use, using electrical equipment more wisely, and increasing your distance from equipment that needs to be powered through the night. Carefully consider the location of any new home before you make an offer. If it's near power lines, a substation, or in a place where the earth's magnetic field is distorted, then it's not a good deal – regardless of the perks it may offer.

Location, Location, Location

Electromagnetic fields typically get weaker as you increase the distance from their source, so choosing a home at least a kilometre from transmission lines and 100 metres from distribution lines ensures lower baseline levels inside the home.

With the move towards solar panels and wind energy, it may be tempting to locate panels above bedrooms with the right sun exposure, place inverters near bedrooms, and position wind turbines out of sight at the back of the house. Before installing any new source of electromagnetic fields, consider its proximity to the bedrooms; remember that EMFs are not deterred by walls, floors, or ceilings.

A badly-located electric panel ensures that all the power to this house passes just above the sleeper's head.

Photo:
Angela Hobbs

Moving appliances and gadgets further from the head of the bed reduces the electromagnetic fields that can disturb your sleep. Remember to include appliances and gadgets on the other side of the wall, floor or ceiling as these often create the strongest EMFs.

Turn Off Power at the Electric Panel

Limiting the nighttime power circulating in the bedroom walls reduces the electromagnetic fields in the bedroom and discourages it as a location for recharging phones and other gadgets during the night.

Identifying which circuits to turn off at night usually takes daylight and two people. First, turn on everything in the house, then have one person work his way through each circuit on the electric panel while the other person reports which circuits were affected. She can then label the circuit appropriately. At bedtime, a selection of circuits can be turned off. Some people may want to turn off everything except the furnace, freezer, fridge, and a bathroom light, while others will turn off power just to the bedrooms.

"Demand switches" offer a convenient alternative to turning off circuits; they only allow electricity to flow to a particular circuit when an appliance on the circuit is turned on. Unfortunately, demand switches cost around $250 US and each electric circuit has to have its own.

Unplug

Unplugging gadgets and transformers eliminate them as sources of electromagnetic fields during the night. These units can usually be recharged earlier in the day when the electromagnetic fields are less inclined to interfere with sleep.

Surge protectors and transformers create their own electromagnetic fields through the night, even if the appliance or gadget at the end of them isn't being used. Many of the electromagnetic fields created by transformers, surge protectors, and rechargers can be eliminated by unplugging them at night (just toggling them off won't do). Unplugging the extra length of wire

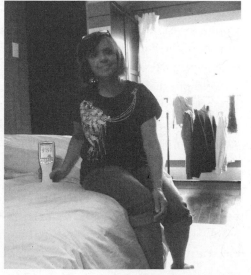

With a Gauss meter identifying the magnetic fields on her pillow, Sandy's persuaded to turn off some of her equipment at night.

Photo:
Angela Hobbs

eliminates any electromagnetic fields created by electricity that's moving to and fro down the wire with nowhere to go and setting up an antenna effect. This "stand-by electricity" accounts for about 10 percent of total residential electricity consumption — about the same amount we expect to save by replacing incandescent lights with compact fluorescent light bulbs.[13] But unplugging appliances that aren't in use reduces electromagnetic fields as well as saving energy, while replacing incandescent light bulbs with compact fluorescent light bulbs may save energy, but also adds strong electromagnetic fields.

Distance

Appliances and gadgets that simply have to run through the night should be located at least six feet from the head of the bed, whether in the same room, an adjacent room, or directly above or below. These might include carbon monoxide detectors, transformers, the electric panel, fridges, freezers, water softeners and furnaces. In these situations, consider moving either the bed or the appliance to maximize the distance between it and the head of the bed.

Summary

The trail of respect for electromagnetic fields winds all the way back to Stone Age peoples, who discovered there were certain easily identifiable land patches that held special powers. With the gradual shift from "history of place" to "history of chronological events," much of the knowledge that would have protected North Americans and Europeans from the health impact of the Earth's stronger magnetic fields was lost, leaving many more people plagued with its associated health issues than necessary.

Without that recognition the stage was set for the AC system to gain a monopoly over power distribution — a monopoly that left the DC system and the battery underdeveloped. In the short term not developing the two systems in parallel resulted in a huge web of powerlines and the rise of new industrial areas. In the longer term it meant that, despite all our efforts to become 'wireless', we would remain tethered to our wall sockets. The need to re-charge an ever-increasing range of equipment surrounds us with multiple layers of EMFs and all the health risks they bring with them. Many of those health risks can be mitigated by simply turning our electrical equipment off when we're not using it.

7 — Skin Contact Chemicals

Tackling the chemicals encumbering your sleep

We're probably all familiar with the advertisements where a beautiful woman with flawless skin slowly smoothes a rich, fragrant lotion down her arms and legs. Maybe that lotion will stop her from itching, maybe it will soothe her sunburn, and maybe it will stop her ageing. But what about all the other things it will do? The advertisement doesn't mention those.

Like all the other unseen, unheard, unfelt, tasteless, and odourless exposures in our bedrooms, the chemicals we come into contact with can damage us. Our skin has evolved to be maximally protective by day and minimally protective at night, when we normally don't do things that are likely to hurt us. A minimally protective skin is extremely vulnerable to the chemicals that reach it. At night those chemicals include phthalates, Bisphenol A, flame retardants and others — chemicals that provide products with desirable characteristics like their texture, dyeability, water or flame resistance, but that can migrate through your skin with harmful effects.

In this chapter you'll meet Chen and see just how vulnerable the skin can be to these chemicals. You'll see what Chen did to reduce that vulnerability and how that vulnerability is used to advantage by drug and cosmetics companies. We'll take a look at where the chemicals we're in contact with through the night came from and how they became such an integral part of the average bedroom. We'll look at how the skin's nighttime vulnerability is used therapeutically and why scientists are concerned about the overdose levels most of us are prone to.

Chen's Story

Chen and his wife had been married for five years, and lived with their four-year-old daughter in a comfortable house in the suburbs. From the day they'd met they'd talked about having a large family, but since the birth of their daughter, the months had passed with no sign of Katy having any siblings. After three years, the young couple finally consulted a fertility clinic and Chen was distraught to find that his ability to father children was in question.

Chen had clearly been fertile during the first year of his marriage, so what had changed? The doctor didn't have an answer for him. In an almost throwaway comment, he suggested it might have something to do with Chen's environment, before laying out several options for him and his wife to consider. Each option seemed more expensive than the last and the young couple knew that if they spent that much money getting pregnant, there'd be nothing left to take care of Katy and her little brother or sister.

The doctor's throwaway comment bothered Chen. He tried repeatedly to think about the things that might have changed since that first year of marriage. Obviously having a daughter now was different — but it meant he got more exercise, ate better, and stuck to a predictable routine. The fact that they now owned a house was different — but not in any bad way; he could afford to redecorate it in the latest trend. Being slightly older was different — but it just meant that he was more confident at work. As far as Chen could see, some things were different, but they were all good.

Then one day Chen's friend, who knew of his fertility struggle, read a magazine article at the dentist's office. "Chen, you should call this woman! She helps people figure out if something in their homes is contributing to their health problems." By the end of the conversation, Chen was convinced to give me a try.

"I've never really worked with anyone whose starting point is infertility," I said. "But I can have a look at your house, tell you what I see, and give you some thoughts."

A week later I was standing in Chen's bedroom. As I'd suspected, the sheets, quilt, pillow, and pajamas were all polyester. The ensuite bathroom, with the shower he used every night, was stacked with shampoos, body washes, soaps, conditioners, and moisturizers. Washable walls and the very best laminated furniture completed the picture. As I surveyed these phthalate-rich surroundings, I asked Chen if he'd been using all these products and sleeping in a polyester bed before he got married.

"No," he said. "I lived with my parents and they only had very old cotton sheets; they didn't have a lot of money. All of the kids shared the same bottle of shampoo and we only had one bathroom for six people. It was usually too busy to have more than one shower in a week. I live in real luxury compared to then."

What Chen Did

After I explained to Chen why I wasn't sure that this really was "luxury" and that his surroundings were filled with environmental estrogens that could be contributing to his infertility, he agreed to make a few simple changes. He would only shower in the morning, keep the products he used and stored in the bathroom to a minimum, and would replace his sheets, pillowcase, quilt, pajamas, and underwear with cotton, for the next six months.

Four months later, I got a call from a very excited young couple. Chen's semen count was up, up high enough that the doctor was confident they would soon conceive.

Contact Chemical Pollution

Where Did It Come From?

Much of our nightly skin contact with chemicals comes from the moisturizers and creams we apply, the detergent and softener residues of incomplete laundering, and the synthetic bedding that surrounds us as we sleep.

Today, almost any item that used to be made from wood, cotton, wool, or metal can be made from plastic. The gradual replacement of products made

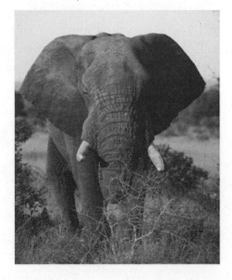

The first plastics grew out of the desire for a more accessible source of ivory

Photo:
iStockphoto

99

from natural materials with those made from synthetic materials began early in the twentieth century. Ivory, used for piano keys, hand-carved ornaments, cutlery handles, and jewellery, was among the first. The market readily accepted the much cheaper and more accessible "celluloid" imitation of elephant and rhino tusks, the production of which proved lucrative for its manufacturers. It didn't take long before other synthetic materials appeared. "Bakelite," considered the first plastic, appeared in 1907 after its inventor, Leo Hendrik Baekeland, found a way of dealing with the foam produced from the phenol and formaldehyde reaction. It was a brittle and expensive product but strong, fire-resistant, and with the excellent insulating characteristics that phenol plastics are still known for.

Polyester sleepwear, sheets, and blankets, exposes us to the same harmful phthalates as those in plastic drink bottles.

Illustration: *"Sweet Sleep" by Chris Hobbs*

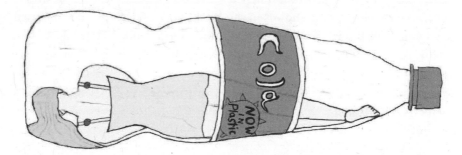

Other plastics arrived during the course of the twentieth century. They offered a level of flexibility their "natural" predecessors couldn't match and the market grew rapidly. Polystyrene quickly gained popularity as Styrofoam. Polyvinyl chloride found a place as shrink wrap and as a substitute for plumbing pipes, and polyamides soon flattered the legs of millions of women as nylons. Spandex, with its capacity to stretch by 600 percent[1] and still recover its shape, was a delight, especially to athletes.

The real boom in plastics came with the outbreak of the Second World War. New opportunities presented themselves with the need for parachutes, radar cable insulation, rubber alternatives, and aircraft canopies. Nylon's light weight and durability made it perfect for parachutes; polyethylene was an ideal insulator for cables; and acrylic glass (better known as Perspex) could be molded into shatterproof aircraft canopies. The war saw the development of polyethylene terephthalate (PET) that would later become the most common plastic used to make polyester fabric and the corrosive resistant beverage containers used for carbonated beverages and acidic fruit juices.

Amongst the more successful developments there were a couple of major slip-ups, many of them related to the highly flammable and explosive nitrocellulose rayon. Production was brought to an end when stories began to circulate of billiard balls exploding mid-game on billiard tables; several candlelit dinners came to an abrupt end with nitrocellulose evening gowns going up in flames.

Where Did It Go?

By the end of World War II, the plastics industry was well established and a major employer. But without military contracts, it faced an uncertain future unless it could identify new markets and reinvent its products to suit them. That need drove the development of new manufacturing techniques that could produce a wide range of products. It also drove the search for new "property-enhancing" chemicals to make the plastic softer, the nail varnish more chip-resistant, and the moisturizer smoother and better penetrating. Chemists competed to create anything that would make fragrances more stable, make medicine capsules release their drug more predictably, and give cleaning products an edge over the competition.

With a little tinkering, chemists were able to respond to the need for new synthetic chemicals and keep up with manufacturers' demands as they pushed their way into the marketplace, idealizing plastic as the ultimate cost-effective product. Between the 1950s and 2007, the demand for plastic rose from five million tons to 230 million tons. By 2010 it exceeded 300 million tons. In the first ten years of the twenty-first century, we've produced almost as much plastic as we did in the whole of the twentieth century.[2]

People were so enthralled by the qualities of these new materials that little thought was given to the possible impacts of the synthetic chemicals. And as long as those plastics were used as substitutes for wood and metal, they weren't all that dangerous. We weren't spending several hours a day with them pressed against our skin. But once plastic became flexible enough to be spun into a weavable thread that could produce a wearable fabric, the danger posed by those chemicals became much greater – now they were in contact with our skin for hours at a time, day and night.

In the production of polyester, the first fibres produced by polyethylene terephthalate (PET) are inflexible and resistant to pigments and dyes. Adding more phthalates after the initial reaction stage makes the fibres more flexible and dyeable. This second batch of phthalates isn't bound to the fibre and disturbs the fibres' structure to the point that even those phthalates that were bound regain their freedom.[3] With this freedom, they migrate to any moist surface — the liquid surrounded by PET bottles, the food surrounded by PET-lined cans, and our skin surrounded by PET clothing, PET bedding, and PET body lotions.

The 1990s saw some research into the ability of phthalates to migrate from polyester fabric onto and into the skin and the impact they had once they arrived. Around the same time, Ahmed Shafik became deeply involved with the World Health Organization's efforts to find a cheap form of contraception for the developing world. Aware that polyester could decrease sperm counts, he began dressing dogs up in a range of underwear made from polyester. After two years of watching his dogs wander around in their fancy pants, Shafik found the dogs' sperm counts had dropped to levels well below those required for conception. Once the pants came off, the dogs' sperm counts returned to normal.

Shafik went on to work with human couples who agreed to participate in his studies. When the men wore the polyester scrotal sacks he provided,[4] their sperm counts dropped. Then he instructed them to stop using the sacks, saw their sperm counts return to normal, awaited the news that they had conceived successfully, and anticipated the fame only the man who'd discovered such a simple method of birth control would warrant.

But though the polyester had temporarily reduced the gentlemen's sperm counts, and although they went on to father children, Shafik's research seems to have come to an abrupt end. There was no fame awaiting Shafik as he emerged from his laboratory, and no one seems to have taken his research to the next level.

What seems to have been a very abrupt halt to this promising research may be related to the chlorine industry's need to protect itself and its market. The plastics industry is one of the few reliable destinations for chlorine gas, which is a by-product of the production of caustic soda. Although there is no shortage of markets for caustic soda — it's used by the paper, soap, detergent, petroleum, and gas scrubbing industries — it's always been more difficult to dispose of chlorine gas, another by-product.

The gas is difficult to store, so unless there is a buyer for it, caustic soda production grinds to a halt.

When Rachel Carson's influential book *Silent Spring* was published in 1962, the chlorine industry began to lose several of its key chlorine gas clients — among them the pesticide, refrigerant, solvent, and pulp-bleaching industries. But thanks to the polyester and plastics industry's ever-increasing demand for chlorine gas, the chlorine industry was just getting back on its feet and investing $130 million a year to reassure its markets and the public[5] when the link between plastics and infertility surfaced in the 1990s.

As the research mounted and the link between plastics and hormone disruption strengthened, the plastics industry was quick to counter the "positive effect" studies with "no effect" studies – a result they ensured by using a specially-bred strain of mice that's insensitive to estrogen.[6]

Today, polyester fabric is used to make boxers, pyjamas, bras, bedding, and a whole range of clothing. Much of that clothing is worn through the night against the warmest parts of the body with the highest penetration rates. As the plastics industry has grown, sperm counts have dropped to about 50 percent of what they were in the 1940s. Poor semen quality is responsible for about half of the infertility amongst couples who seek help from fertility clinics.[7] When couples do eventually conceive, high phthalate levels in the mother affect their offspring's ability to have children.

The Dose and the Overdose

The Dose – Contact Chemicals as Therapy

As medical researchers have explored alternative ways to deliver drugs and medicines, the skin has become a subject of considerable research. Being able to deliver drugs through the skin has many advantages. It eliminates much of the fear and pain of injections, it reduces the need for complicated designs required for medicines that pass through the digestive tract, it allows pain medications to be applied close to the area where relief is needed, and it lends itself to periodic release over longer periods of time.

To develop the right medicines, scientists needed to know which areas of the body were more and less penetrable, whether there were times of the day when penetration speed changed, and whether certain areas tended to be more acidic or warmer. The research drove the highly specific

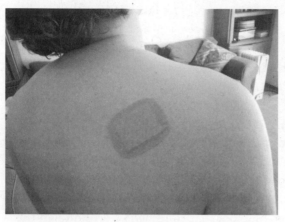

Transdermal patches exploit the skin's vulnerability to deliver medication

Photo:
Angela Hobbs

design of today's transdermal patches and creams: put them on your forehead when they're designed for your feet, and the medication will penetrate about twice as fast as it should.[8] Put them on damaged or dry skin, and the penetration will be significantly faster. Put them in areas with a greater concentration of hair follicles, and the medication is likely to penetrate even faster because the hair follicles act as shunt routes that, along with sweat glands, increase the skin's surface area.

The medical professions haven't been the only ones interested in the skin's peculiarities. Cosmetics companies have been equally eager to develop products that exploit the skin barrier's regular nighttime weakening. They know that every night, at around eight o'clock, the skin's water content begins to drop and continues to decline until about three in the morning. This period when the skin's water content and barrier recovery are at their lowest is the time of least resistance to the penetration of chemicals and micro-organisms. It's the time when moisturizers work best.[9]

The Overdose — Contact Chemicals as a Health Risk

Plastics were originally used to replace wood and metal. Once they developed enough to replace cotton and wool in clothing, people who wore them began experiencing new symptoms. These drove the search for a wider range of "moisturizers" and a broader range of synthetic chemicals. As cancers of the skin became more prevalent than cancers in any other organ,[10] sun exposure was fingered as the culprit rather than the multiple layers of unbound chemicals in regular contact with the skin during the night.

That constant exposure to unbound environmental estrogens reduces testosterone levels in men[11] and lowers their sperm count and fertility. In women, environmental estrogens increase overall estrogen levels.[12] That's okay during the day — estrogen is supposed to be high then. That's when it's working to maintain the skin's protective barrier, speed its healing, and stifle osteoporosis and cardiovascular disease.[13] But estrogen levels should be low at night. Exposure to these chemicals at night cranks up estrogen levels, which distracts melatonin from its proper sleep role, because another of melatonin's roles is to keep estrogens levels low.[14]

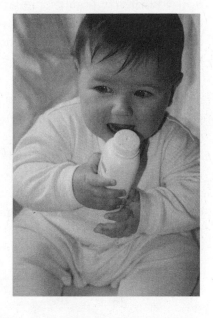

Phthalates from powders, shampoos and other personal care products persist in the body for twenty-four hours after they're applied

Photo:
Nicola Gilbert

Several other chemicals, each with its own health impact, gain access through the skin and into the body thanks to the penetration-enhancing characteristics of phthalates. These chemicals are also added to fabrics and personal care products after the initial reaction, leaving them unbound and eager to migrate. As the body heats up and polyester fabrics trap moisture against the skin, these chemicals are ensured an easy passage right into the skin.

Bisphenol A (BPA) is used to make water-repellent food containers, lotions, face creams, bedding, fibrefill pillows, and fabrics. The concerns about it are centred on its widespread prevalence, its ability to increase estrogen levels, its impact on male fertility,[15] and its stimulation of the cytokines implicated in allergies and asthmas.[16] A 2005 study by the American-based Centers for Disease Control found detectable levels of BPA in 95 percent of the 400 adults they tested. Canadian levels are similar.[17]

Isocyanates are used in the production of polyurethane mattresses and mattress pads. They play a role in asthma, and for a long time their access to the lungs was thought to be limited to breathing. Much of the research into the relationship between isocyanates and asthma has been done in workplaces where isocyanates and asthma levels were both high.

But even after the workplaces were cleaned up and ventilation was improved the asthma remained. Initially bewildered researchers eventually realized that, like peanuts and latex, isocyanates can set off a reaction in the lungs even though they gain access through the skin. Today the skin is thought to be a more significant entry point for isocyanates than the lungs.[18]

Brominated Flame Retardants (BFRs) are added to foams and other products to slow the speed of burning. A good third of a foam's weight can be made up of BFRs.[19] Bras padded with estrogen-mimicking BFRs may be contributing to the elevated levels of BFRs in the breast milk of Canadian women[20], and to breast cancer rates.

About 75 different types of BFRs make up the 200,000 tons produced every year.[21] Asia, who exports many of her products to the west, uses over half of them and shows a distinct preference for tetrabromoisphenol A (TBBPA). Like Bisphenol A, it raises estrogen levels at all the wrong times and inhibits the T-cells that defend the body against bacteria and viruses.[22] The Americas use about a third of those 200,000 tons and prefer polybrominated diphenyl ethers (PBDE). PBDEs are known to disrupt thyroid hormones and the brain's neurons, affecting learning, memory and behaviour.[23]

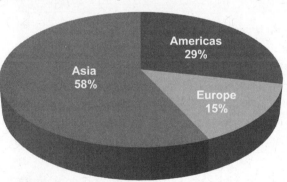

Asia uses more than its fair share of brominated flame retardants, but much of it is to make products for export

Parabens are used to preserve body lotions, shampoos, conditioners, sunscreen, antiperspirants, deodorants, colognes, perfumes, and soaps. Like Bisphenol A, they raise estrogen levels at all the wrong times, making unnecessary demands on the melatonin that contains them through the night.

Triclosan is used widely as an antibacterial and antimicrobial in socks, underpants, bedding, soaps, deodorants, mouthwashes, and acne medications. This potent product takes no prisoners: whether the bacteria in question are friendly (like those involved in digestion) or unfriendly (like those that make us sick), it kills them all.

Sodium Lauryl Sulphate (SLS) is a degreaser added to detergents, bubble baths, shampoos, and body washes. Its tendency to strip the skin of its protective oily layer reduces the skin's efficiency as a barrier against chemicals and bacteria.

Dealing with Skin Contact Chemicals

The Main Concern

The main concern with the chemicals that come into contact with the skin during the night is that they unnecessarily distract melatonin, reducing the quantity that's left to perform other tasks and thereby contributing to the sleep/wake conflict. Figure 7 shows a selection of studies into the sleep and health impact that can have. Polyester sets up transdermal patch-like conditions, trapping moisture and releasing the phthalates that encourage other chemicals to penetrate the skin. These conditions trigger the rise of estrogen and the distraction of melatonin as it struggles to contain these surging levels.

A good deal of media attention has focused on how we ingest phthalates by drinking water from PET bottles, but there's been far less interest in the phthalates that migrate into our skin. Unless you develop an obvious reaction, you may be oblivious to this danger.

This exposure is all the more worrisome because anything close to your skin for eight hours at a time, night after night, can have a cumulative effect. Even if you don't apply body lotion every night, you or your family members may still use fabric softener on your sheets, wear cute little polyester pyjamas, sleep between polyester sheets and/or on polyurethane foam mattresses, or sleep in a polyester bra.

Addressing the Concern

The concern can usually be addressed by replacing fabrics that come into contact with the skin at night with natural alternatives, barricading the chemicals in materials that can't be replaced, minimizing the use of creams and lotions before bed, and bathing in the morning rather than the evening.

Fig. 7 — The Health Impact of Contact Chemicals[24]

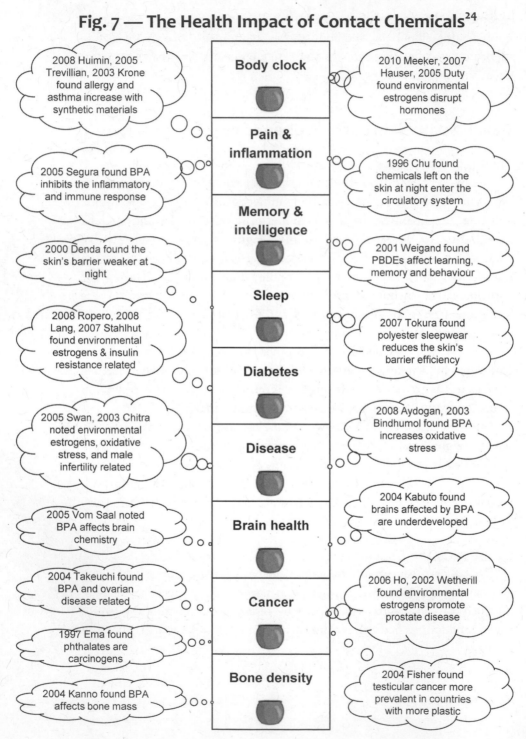

2008 Huimin, 2005 Trevillian, 2003 Krone found allergy and asthma increase with synthetic materials

2005 Segura found BPA inhibits the inflammatory and immune response

2000 Denda found the skin's barrier weaker at night

2008 Ropero, 2008 Lang, 2007 Stahlhut found environmental estrogens & insulin resistance related

2005 Swan, 2003 Chitra noted environmental estrogens, oxidative stress, and male infertility related

2005 Vom Saal noted BPA affects brain chemistry

2004 Takeuchi found BPA and ovarian disease related

1997 Ema found phthalates are carcinogens

2004 Kanno found BPA affects bone mass

Body clock

Pain & inflammation

Memory & intelligence

Sleep

Diabetes

Disease

Brain health

Cancer

Bone density

2010 Meeker, 2007 Hauser, 2005 Duty found environmental estrogens disrupt hormones

1996 Chu found chemicals left on the skin at night enter the circulatory system

2001 Weigand found PBDEs affect learning, memory and behaviour

2007 Tokura found polyester sleepwear reduces the skin's barrier efficiency

2008 Aydogan, 2003 Bindhumol found BPA increases oxidative stress

2004 Kabuto found brains affected by BPA are underdeveloped

2006 Ho, 2002 Wetherill found environmental estrogens promote prostate disease

2004 Fisher found testicular cancer more prevalent in countries with more plastic

Replacing

Bedding alternatives usually include either pure or blended: linen, cotton, hemp, wool, soy, and bamboo. Organic varieties are less likely to have been treated with chemical washes, dyes, toxins or pesticides, but they can be pricey. Pillow alternatives to polyester include: rubber, shredded rubber, and down. Mattress alternatives include cotton futons and possibly latex. Although cotton was once a crop that required heavy pesticide use, most cotton today is genetically modified, greatly reducing the concern over pesticide residues.

Barricading

A thick layer of a natural fabric can be used to create a barrier between the sleeper and the chemicals in pillows and mattresses. Wrapping foam mattresses in heavy cotton bedspreads or adding a couple of extra pillowcases to the pillow will usually create an adequate barrier to migrating chemicals.

Minimizing Nighttime Use of Creams and Lotions

The skin is most vulnerable to the chemicals in lotions and creams between 8 p.m. and 3 a.m. The skin is more effective at keeping harmful chemicals from penetrating into the bloodstream during the day — which means it's probably much safer to apply those potions in the morning.

There are often safer product alternatives. Skin Deep offers an online searchable database at www.cosmeticsdatabase.com that ranks products based on the safety of their ingredients. It allows you to search for products you use frequently, and tells you what's in them and what's in the alternatives.

As the dangers of hormone-disrupting chemicals gain recognition, the nascent green chemical industry, with its focus on less environmentally damaging chemicals and support of chemical alternatives like genetic modification, is likely to grow. Its focus today tends to be on alternative food packaging and cleaning products, but as government regulations increasingly limit the use of phthalates and environmental concerns continue to rise, green chemicals will have opportunities to expand into new areas, and will probably move in quickly.

Summary

The tsunamic growth of plastic and synthetic chemical industries has been accompanied by an alarming rise in conditions provoked by environmental estrogens: cancers, bone fractures, infertility, and the like. The skin can't evolve its protective routine fast enough to keep up with the chemical assaults that are part of life in the twenty-first century.

With so many new chemicals arriving on the scene at the same time, identifying which of them was responsible for the hormone disruptions provoking ill health was challenging — a challenge often compounded by researchers' need to sustain their funding — they have mortgages to pay, too. By testing the chemicals individually, even though their impact was known to result from combinations, and working with creatures known not to exhibit the symptoms being tested for, researchers ensured the "no effects" results their funders wanted!

There is still a growing demand for products that make our lives easier and more luxurious, but the news that almost half of the product might be phthalates often falls on deaf ears. Along with requirements for multiple proofs, slow recalls from store shelves, and the widespread acceptance of manipulated research, the stage has been set for the continued influx of hormone-disrupting chemicals into our daily lives.

Though scientists have made use of the skin's natural rhythms for transdermal drug delivery, we're only vaguely conscious of the impact the unbound chemicals surrounding it at night can have. These chemicals prolong the skin's weakened state, enhance the penetration of other chemicals, increase estrogen levels, and generally distract melatonin from the real jobs it should be doing — giving us sound sleep and health. Until the green chemical industry catches this wave, you should reduce your nightly contact with chemicals by cautiously choosing fabrics and materials, carefully selecting personal care products, and thorough laundering.

8 — Air Pollutants and Air Ions

Managing the air pollutants hampering your sleep

Air pollutants come at us from all directions. We may live near an industrial plant, a landfill site, or a dry cleaner that fills the air with pollutants day and night, or we may depend on chemical air fresheners and fragrances to keep our air "fresh." In this chapter, we'll look at how the ions in the synthetic furnishings around us interfere with the air's natural self-cleaning mechanism, how the growing threat of bioterrorism has helped us understand just what's going on in the air around us, and how we can use that new information to our advantage. But first I'd like you to meet Jenny and witness her struggle with air pollutants.

Jenny's Story

Like many nocturnal asthma sufferers, Jenny tended to suffer attacks at around 4 a.m.[1] She wasn't at all sure that her doctor's diagnosis was right. She'd never had any trouble breathing and she took good care of herself. She'd never smoked, got plenty of exercise and fresh air, and ate a diet rich in fruit and vegetables. If this really was asthma, why did it only strike at night? Wouldn't it have hit her during one of her vigorous mountain bike rides? She dutifully took the medication her doctor offered, but was convinced that mold in her house was at the root of her problem.

In the hope that I would be able to locate the elusive mold she'd been searching for during the last two years, Jenny set up an appointment for us to meet at the house where she lived with her husband and their two teenage sons — a two-storey home on a busy road.

Jenny had first noticed the mold problem about two years earlier. "I can't really smell it," she said. "The air just feels wrong, so I know it's there." Jenny had looked everywhere for her mold. She'd taken portions of drywall off her basement walls, she'd checked behind the tiles in the bathroom, she'd even looked for it in the seal between the kitchen sink and counter — but she hadn't yet found any trace of mold. She'd had all the metal ducts sprayed with an antibacterial product, but that didn't get rid of it either.

"I know it's here," she declared, "but I just can't find it, so I need you to find it for me before I end up destroying all the walls in my house!"

Jenny walked me through her house, pointing out all the places where she'd looked for mold, and where she'd sprayed bleach, just in case. I checked other obvious places, like the space below the showers that builders often leave hollow and can harbor ideal mold conditions if the shower leaks, but there was no suggestion that there was mold, or the damp conditions it loves, anywhere in her house.

What did strike me, though, was that on such a beautifully warm day, all the windows were closed. Jenny explained that she kept all the windows closed all the time to prevent the road pollution from entering her house. During the summer, the air conditioner circulated cool air, and during the winter the furnace circulated warm air. So, in effect, all the air in her house passed through treated metal ducts all year round.

The upper floor of the house was divided into three bedrooms. The boys each had a room and shared a bathroom. Their bedrooms faced the back of the house and their doors were kept closed because they insisted on sleeping with open windows. These two carpeted rooms each had a large wooden desk, bureau, cotton bedding, and heavy cotton curtains. The master bedroom at the front of the house faced the busy street and had an expansive ensuite bathroom with no door. The furnishings in this room were all synthetic. On the laminated wood floor stood a bureau and bed frame made of laminated plywood. The bedding and curtains were polyester. Plastic storage boxes stood floor to ceiling in the wardrobe.

Jenny looked at me in disbelief when I asked her if she'd ever tried sleeping in the living room or one of the boys' bedrooms.

"I want you to help me find the **mold**," she replied, with major stress on the word "mold."

"I understand that, Jenny, really I do," I replied, "but part of tracking the source of the mold is to identify the air currents carrying it. Since you're the one who's sensitive to it, I'd like to suggest that we use you as our canary and test a couple of areas in the house by getting you to sleep there."

What I wanted to say was, "Jenny, any mold problem you may have is insignificant compared to the drastically ion-depleted air you're creating here. The first thing we need to do is demonstrate that you can sleep, symptom-free, in some places so that we can open your mind to the possibility there are other things wrong with your air."

I managed to persuade Jenny to spend the coming week's nights in one of her sons' rooms. When we met up again, she was pleased to report that she hadn't had a single breathless night. She found it totally confusing that she could sleep better with the pollution and mold coming in through an open window than when the windows were shut. This was great, we were making headway, I thought. Jenny had been reminded that what she was really looking for was relief from the early morning asthma, not mold. Mold had simply become the fixation of her search for relief. Now it was time to take out my ion meter and show her the difference in the ion levels between the room where she'd slept well and the room that provoked the almost nightly attacks. The meter confirmed my suspicions: the master bedroom readings were negligible, while the son's bedroom was within the "normal" range.

Jenny was very curious about the numbers she was seeing. She wanted to know what the meter was counting and why it was able to count so many more of them in her son's room than in her room. Until now, the only thing she'd ever considered was mold, and all of her actions had been in response to that limited understanding of what was in her air.

Now Jenny seemed ready to understand more about her air, and so I explained what her surroundings and habits were doing to it. On the one hand, the metal ducts of her ventilation system, the closed windows, the purely synthetic finishes, and plastic storage containers were keeping her air ions – nature's air cleaners — at very low levels. And on the other hand, those synthetic surfaces, the cleaning products she used in her mold battles, and the range of cosmetics and toiletries in her doorless ensuite bathroom were putting chemicals into her air. Without air ions to weigh them down, dropping them to the floor where they could be vacuumed up, these chemicals remained airborne. As she breathed this air into her lungs, the chemicals irritated them, causing nitric oxide levels to rise and start an asthma attack.

What Jenny Did

Once Jenny understood what was going on in her air, all the energy she'd invested in mold shifted to ions. Within a couple of days, she'd increased the ion level in her bedroom to normal and moved back in. She started by getting her sons to help her carry the bureau and all the plastic storage boxes down into the basement. They brought up an old wooden bureau that had seen better days. Next, she installed doors on her bathroom and wardrobe. These she shut at night before getting into bed. She took out many of the products and cleaners in her bathroom, even though the door would stop them entering her nighttime air. She started leaving the boys' bedroom doors open at night so that she and her husband could benefit from the fresher night air and ions that filled their rooms. Their bed gained a cotton bed skirt and bedding, and they replaced their polyester sleepwear with cotton.

When I checked on Jenny a few weeks later, she hadn't had a single asthma attack and was sleeping well night after night.

Air Pollution

Where Did It Come From?

It's fairly common to think of air pollution as something outside the home that someone else is paid to deal with. It might be the gas stack flare at the local oil refinery spewing sulphur dioxide when the day's winds are too low to carry the rotten-egg smell away. It may be the diesel school bus idling for an hour because the driver doesn't have time to go home and it's too cold not to have the engine running. It may be the winds that have carried the smoke from the distant forest fire right to your front door, or it may be a poorly installed air intake to your ventilation system that fills your house with the fragrance of your neighbour's fabric softener.

Typically, air pollution is something we're alerted to when something smells different, when the smoke detector whistles, the carbon monoxide sensor alerts us, or we discover that our neighbour is installing radon vents. Yet, in much of the developed world, the air inside our homes is far more polluted than the air outside — often at least **five times** more. And we may not even be able to smell it.

Much of that pollution comes from normal activities inside our homes: cooking, cleaning, bathing, laundry, and hobby activities. A good deal of it comes from synthetic items like furniture, flooring, curtains, clothing, upholstery, carpets, and storage containers. And a great deal comes from the warm plastic casings and innards of computers, televisions, and other technology.

We've welcomed synthetic products into our homes for many reasons. They're usually cheaper and less flammable than products made of natural materials. They come in colours that lend themselves to coordination with the existing décor; they aren't attractive to moths (insects know better!); and they offer relatively easy maintenance. You can easily wipe the spilt coffee from a laminated end table where a wooden one might be permanently ruined.

As with the products we learned about in chapter 7, the qualities that make synthetic furniture and furnishings so attractive are created with chemicals — chemicals that are usually added too late in the manufacturing process to become "bound." So once that product takes its place hanging from the curtain or clothes rail, supporting or encasing the television, completing the entertainment system, or adding a touch of sophistication to the bedroom, those unbound chemicals prepare to migrate — right into the warmed or cooled air we're usually working so hard to keep in our homes.

Starting with the oil crisis of the 1970s, homes and workplaces have become more and more energy-efficient. Many workplaces seem hermetically sealed; ventilation systems may deliver only five of the fifteen cubic feet of air that they used to deliver for each person. At home, homeowners would rather live with "a little mustiness" than open the windows and watch their hard-earned income (in the form of warmed or air-conditioned air) disappear. These tightly sealed homes, the ever-increasing availability of new technology, the prevalence of synthetic materials, and an endless supply of fragranced products are at the root of many of the air quality problems faced by home owners. The most common air quality disruptors are phthalates, brominated flame retardants, formaldehyde, toluene, radon, mold, bacteria, ozone, and carbon monoxide. Others like lead and mercury are reappearing with the increasing use of printers, televisions, computers, and other electronic equipment in bedrooms.

Phthalates enter the bedroom as products made from plastic and polyvinyl chloride. These products include shower curtains, tablecloths, furniture, wall coverings, adhesives, paint, computer shells, television casings, storage boxes, shower stalls, and cosmetics. Heat from a shower, bath, television program, or computer session increases the phthalate migration from the products.

Brominated flame retardants enter the bedroom on materials that need to be resistant to fire. These products include the circuit boards, components, cables, and plastic covers of electronics equipment, but, ironically, heat speeds their migration from these products. Once they're out in a darkened bedroom, away from the sunlight that could speed their breakdown, they can persist for a very long time, with the result that they're much more common indoors than outside.

Formaldehyde enters the bedroom as a preservative in cosmetics, cleaners, permanent press finishes, furniture, and furnishings. The heat-resistant phenol formaldehyde used in adhesives, paints, laminates, particleboard, and plywood can be problematic. It's associated with environmental sensitivities, watery eyes, burning sensations, and nausea.

Toluene enters the bedroom in paints, sealants, adhesives, disinfectants, and in toluene diisocyanate, which is used in the polyurethane foam of soft furnishings. Toluene shares first place with formaldehyde as the chemical most commonly found in the air of homes. Once in the body, it can affect vigilance, reaction time, and memory. It's particularly harmful to infants because it affects their immature immune systems and makes them more susceptible to illness and disease.[2]

Radon enters homes through cracks and gaps in surfaces exposed to radium- and uranium-rich soils, rocks, and groundwater. This odourless, tasteless, invisible gas emits alpha particles that become a potent source of free radicals when breathed into the lungs.

Radon penetrates homes through cracks and gaps in surfaces that have contact with radon-rich soils and groundwater

Photo:
www.accuraterad onservicesllc.com

Mold enters the bedroom from the air. At any given time there are thousands of different mold spores hanging in the air currents around us.

Occasionally they land in conditions that offer them a constant source of oxygen, food, and moisture, where they'll reproduce unashamedly, forming large, smelly colonies. A mold's toxicity depends on the surface it grows on and its lifecycle stage when water is introduced.[3] A mold growing in soil may be harmless, while the same mold growing on gypsum or wood can provoke alarming reactions.

Bacteria and viruses usually enter homes when the people carrying them sneeze, cough, and breathe. Shared surfaces like telephones, door handles, remote controls for changing television channels, keyboards, towels, taps, and milk and water jug handles, often play an enabling role in the movement of bacteria and viruses between people.

Ozone enters the bedroom as a by-product of high-voltage electrical equipment, including laser printers, photocopiers, ionic air purifiers, and some negative ion generators. It has a bleach-like smell that we don't usually notice until after our eyes have started to itch.

Carbon monoxide enters the bedroom from faulty or poorly maintained combustion systems related to fireplaces, hot water heaters, furnaces, kerosene heaters, gas stoves, and garages. It doesn't smell and can quickly build up to levels that cause headaches, nausea, dizziness, and confusion.

Lead enters the bedroom from the circuit boards and plastic covers of televisions, computers and other electronic equipment. The storage and use of printers, inks and hobby supplies in bedrooms can also contribute. Heat created in this equipment during use encourages the lead to enter the air, often aided by the little fans that prevent the equipment from overheating. Much of a computer's weight is due to the lead used in its circuit boards. During the late twentieth century tremendous efforts were made to reduce the lead in homes because of the impact it has on brain

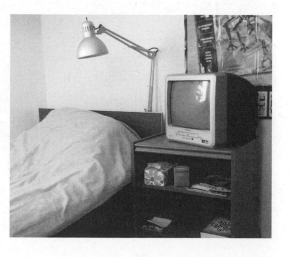

Plastic casings contain unbound chemicals and lead. Heat from the working TV or computer increases their migration into the air

Photo:
Angela Hobbs

development and the learning ability of growing children.

Mercury enters our bedrooms from electronic equipment, hobby supplies, printer inks, batteries, and compact fluorescent light (CFL) bulbs. Because mercury affects learning ability and memory, its use in many products, including the thimerosal preservative used in combined children's vaccinations, has been phased out during the last twenty years.

Where Did It Go?

Traditionally, most of the emphasis on improving the air quality in our homes has targeted the products that pollute it — the cleaners we use to clean it, the furniture we use to make it more comfortable and functional, the machines we use to heat and cool, moisten and dry it. But while we've made inroads using that type of thinking, we haven't been able to even dent the explosive asthma rates that plague the developed world.

More recently, the looming threat of bioterrorism has unleashed research funds that allowed scientists to look at air quality from another angle – how to speed up the removal of pathogens and chemicals from the air. That research has led to a much better understanding of how pollutants become airborne, remain airborne, and break down. These mechanisms revolve around the presence and movements of positive and negative ions in the air.

Crashing waves, showers, and waterfalls fill the air with the ions that clean it and enhance our sense of well-being

***Photo:** Angela Hobbs*

Ions in the air are formed when an electron is forced to leave its atom — often by lightning, moving water, cosmic rays, ultraviolet light, and radioactive minerals in the ground. The solitary electron attaches to a neutral molecule to form a negative ion, while the original atom, bereft of an electron, becomes a positive ion.

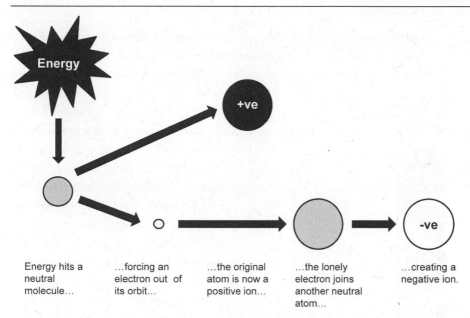

Energy

+ve

-ve

| Energy hits a neutral molecule… | …forcing an electron out of its orbit… | …the original atom is now a positive ion… | …the lonely electron joins another neutral atom… | …creating a negative ion. |

Ions are created when energy strikes a neutral molecule

These ions are carried to our homes on air currents. If those air currents travel across natural terrain, the air arrives with a plentiful supply of ions ready to go to work cleaning the air. Like magnets, they are attracted to anything with an opposite charge. If that's dust, chemicals, or bacteria, they'll ultimately become too heavy to remain airborne; they fall to the floor where they'll eventually be vacuumed up. If the air currents carry them on a journey through a synthetic terrain, full of polluting factories and traffic, and asphalt roads, the air arrives depleted of ions – they will already have been used up. Without a plentiful supply of ions in our air, there's nothing to attract and weigh down pollutants and bacteria, so they remain circulating in our air where we can breathe them.

While much of the air that wafts into our homes is already depleted of ions there's an additional depletion that occurs after it arrives.

Location	Ions/cm^3
Waterfall	1500 - 4000
Lake	1500 - 2500
City	300 - 500
Industrial area	80 - 200
House (closed windows)	60 - 300

Air ions are more plentiful in areas with moving water

Many popular synthetic surfaces in our homes today carry a charge that depletes the air's ion levels even further — the shift from natural to synthetic materials for building and furnishing our homes has seen to that.

LEVEL OF CHARGE	
+	Air
	Human body
	Leather
	Glass
	Quartz
	Mica
	Human hair
	Nylon
	Wool
	Lead
	Silk
	Aluminum
0	Paper
	Cotton
	Steel
	Wood
	Acrylic
	Polystyrene
	Resins
	Nickel, copper
	Brass, silver
	Gold, platinum
	Acetate, rayon
	Synthetic rubber
	Polyester
	Styrene
	Polyurethane
	Polyethylene
−	Polypropylene
	Vinyl (PVC)

The charges of everyday sources.

The air's ion content depends on the strength of the source and what's using it up

Instead of the neutrally-charged whitewash that once covered interior walls, most of today's walls are painted with negatively-charged plastic paints. Instead of carpets woven with positively-charged wool, our floors are covered with negatively-charged polypropylene carpets. Instead of charge-neutral wooden building materials and furniture, we're surrounded by negatively-charged pressed wood, plywood, and laminates. Like magnets that repel a similar charge, the charge in these surfaces repels similarly-charged bacteria and pollutants right back into the air we breathe.

In really good air, like the air you breathe deeply on a summer's day by the lake, there's something like 2000 ions/cm^3 in a negative to positive ratio of about 4:5. Once you leave the lake and start the journey back into town, the quantity of ions in the air takes a tumble. With the windows closed and the air conditioning running full-tilt, many of those ions are sucked out of the air in the car, attracted by their opposites lurking in the synthetic upholstery and other materials. As you drive into the city, with its paved roads, traffic fumes, and miles of concrete and industrial sites, the air's ion content drops again — sometimes to as little as 300 ions/cm^3.

So now you're home, the picnic hamper's unpacked, and you curl up for the evening with a good book. Here, if your furnishings are synthetic, your windows are tightly closed, and your air conditioner is humming passing your air through metal ducts, the ion count in your air will probably drop again — to about 100 ions/cm^3. Chances are you'll be exhausted within the hour and tell yourself that the day spent lazing around at the lake wore you out. It's unlikely that you'll associate that exhaustion with the ion-depleted air in the home that you've returned to.

Most of the synthetic surfaces that are sucking the remaining ions out of our air — like our bookcases, computer casings, pianos, bureaus, bed frames, and lampshades — are also adding pollutants to it through offgassing and cleaning product residues.

The Dose and the Overdose

Dose — Ions as a Therapy

Teachers and parents notice just how difficult it is to keep children focused on windy, stormy days. Changes in the air's ion content can have a significant impact on people without their being fully aware of it, and about a quarter of the population is particularly sensitive.[4] Even Hippocrates (460 BC — 370 BC) mentioned it in his book *On Regimen in Acute Diseases*:

> *"The winds which must pass over mountains to reach cities do not only dry, but also disturb the air which we breathe and the bodies of men so as to engender disease."*

But it wasn't until the 1930s that clinical experiments were set up to explore the relationship between the air's ion content and the physical sensations people experienced. At the time, since they were dealing with air that had a plentiful supply of ions — there were few synthetic products and little pollution depleting the air of its ions, the research focused on the health impact associated with negative or positive ions rather than their combined absence. Friedrich Dessauer was one of those scientists whose curiosity was piqued by people's complaints about mountain winds like the foehn, chinook, sirocco, simoom, Santa Ana, and zonda. He set up an electrostatic generator and tested the reactions of his patients to air laden with positive ions and then negative ones. In the positive air, his patients complained of headaches, dizziness, migraines, depression, and listlessness, but as the air became more negatively charged, those symptoms faded.

Other researchers continued to look at ions until they were able to explain why the mountain winds brought increasing vehicle collisions, work accidents, crime, suicides, homicides, and hospital admissions.[5] Their consensus was that negative ions promote feelings of well-being, improving nerve impulses, mood, and sleep, while positive ions impede nerve impulses, good mood, and sleep.[6]

The research explained why storms and the strong mountain winds have such an impact on the day-to-day well-being of so many people. The air moving hurriedly over land creates friction that produces ions. While the wind blows, the ions form two layers. The positive ions are attracted to the earth by its negative charge, so they stay low, while the negative ions rise, repelled by the earth's negative charge. After the strong winds have passed, the two layers combine again to restore the healthy plentiful and balanced ion supply that makes everyone feel good.

Once the research into the mountain winds had explained the accompanying symptoms, it came to an end. Very little of it continued through the 1960s and beyond, as plastics and synthetic products flooded the market and precipitated a downward spiralling of the ions in our homes. The total lack of recognition of the ion's critical health role was reflected in the spa's move into the local shopping centre. Spas were traditionally health retreats up in the mountains, near waterfalls and beside oceans — places that offered the same healing atmosphere as the famous Belgian town of Spa. Today's North American spas, for the most part, have become synonymous with Botox treatments and toenail clipping; they've lost the healing essence of the traditional version and repeated many of the ion-depleting mistakes of most bedrooms, offices, hospitals, and schools: synthetic furnishings, synthetic flooring, synthetic treatment products, and synthetic cleaning product residues.

Much of the recent interest in air ions has been spurred on by the threat of bioterrorism — if some noxious agent were to be released into our air, how would be able to get it out fast? That research has discovered that an abundant supply of air ions can rapidly and efficiently remove bacteria from hospital air.[7]

Name	Description
Acinetobacter baumannii	A multi-resistant bacteria that causes infections and pneumonia
Aspergillus versicolor	An allergen and irritant
Candida albicans	A bacteria that causes oral and genital infections
Enterococcus malodoratus	A resistant bacteria that causes genital infections
Escherichia coli (E. coli)	A bacteria that causes food poisoning
Mycobacterium parafortuitum	A relatively harmless bacteria
Neurospora crassa	A red bread mold
Penicillium notatum	The bacteria that Alexander Fleming made penicillin from
Pseudomonas aeruginosa	A common increasingly resistant bacteria that causes inflammation
Serratia marcescens	A bacteria that causes infections of the intestines and urinary tract
Staphylococcus albus	A common skin bacteria that can cause infections
Staphylococcus chromogenes	A penicillin-resistant bacteria

These and many other harmful airborne bacteria are reduced when air ions are plentiful

In one experiment, nurses' charge-neutral cotton aprons were switched with negatively-charged plastic ones, this revealed that the spread of infections by the *Acinetobacter* bacteria could be reduced:[8] The negatively-charged bacteria were simply repelled by the negatively-charged aprons, so they didn't get a free ride between wards. In a similar ion-repulsion experiment, researchers found they could reduce infections in intensive care settings by increasing the negative charge on items that came into contact with patients: plastic ventilators, nebulizers, urinary tubes, and surgeons' gloves. In some cases, positive ions in the air were responsible for reducing the bacteria that were circulating, while in others it was the negative air ions.

Today, ion therapy is often used to treat burns. It promotes healing, reduces the pain and infection associated with the burn, and soothes the restlessness that the victims often experience.

Overdose – Air Pollution as a Health Risk

Bad air is being increasingly recognized as the cause of the most common chronic disease amongst children: asthma. Asthma affects more than 300 million people worldwide, kills about 180,000 people every year, and increases by 50 percent every ten years.[9] This kind of increase cannot have a genetic explanation; the time frame is simply too short. There's a distinct possibility that alongside contact chemicals, polluted air plays a role in the development of asthma and other breathing-related health issues.

Overdose situations can develop quickly in homes, and they're often related to the arrival of new furniture, appliances, electronic equipment, clothes, foam products and furnishings. The first year that a new product spends in our homes is usually the period during which unbound chemicals migrate most heavily. Most of us recognize that migration as the "new home" or "new car" smell. During this first year, those products deliver a double punch by contributing pollutants to the air and depleting it of the ions necessary to ensure their removal.

Even after a big-ticket synthetic product has aged and its smell has faded, potential overdose conditions exist in many North American homes, even in products as seemingly innocuous as the laundry soaps and softeners we use. It's rare for these chemicals to be rinsed off once the "cleaning" is done, even though *many of those cleaning products are too toxic to be disposed of at regular landfill sites.* Chemical air fresheners are often added to the mix in an effort to "fix" bad air. Laundry is rarely rinsed adequately and fragranced fabric softeners with long-lasting scents are becoming increasingly common. Wrinkle releasers, perfumed drawer inserts, chemically-fragranced personal care products used during bathing, cooking fumes, hobby solvents, chlorinated water, and a myriad of other chemical sources all add to the chemical stew in the air of the average home.

The prevalence of negatively-charged surfaces and depleted ion levels greatly contributes to the high levels of pollutants and bacteria found in the air in the average home. That combination probably also contributes to the common situation of colds and viruses that travel "right through the house," giving everyone in the family a turn — there's nothing to take them out of the air!

Because their journey to the lungs is so direct, these bacteria and pollutants bypass the detoxification process that kicks in via the digestive system when they get into the body with our food and drink. Once in the lungs, they can cause major irritation and gain access to other parts of the body through the circulatory system.

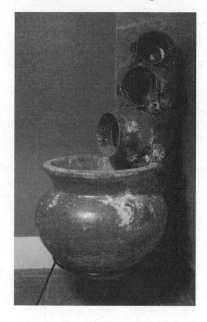

Feng Shui uses cascading water to ensure a plentiful supply of both positive and negative ions

Photo:
Angela Hobbs

Although many people look to ionizers to fix their air, these tend to provide only negative ions. The real problem in most homes is that there are simply too few ions of either charge to rid the air of all we put into it. Feng shui's reliance on cascading water recognizes the importance of a plentiful supply of both.

Dealing with Air Pollutants

The Main Concern
The main concern with air pollutants in the bedroom is that they distract melatonin from the many roles it already has to perform at night. Figure 9 shows a selection of studies into the sleep and health impact that can have. During the third of our lives we spend sleeping, we take a good three thousand of our ten thousand daily breaths. Pollutants that remain airborne in our bedrooms get sucked into the lungs during those breaths. From there they access the rest of the body, without going through any detoxification processes.

Addressing the Concern
We can improve our bedroom air by diluting, reducing, and barricading pollutants. We can also complement this traditional approach by adding charge-neutral surfaces that leave air ions available.

Fig. 9 — The Health Impact of Air Pollutants[10]

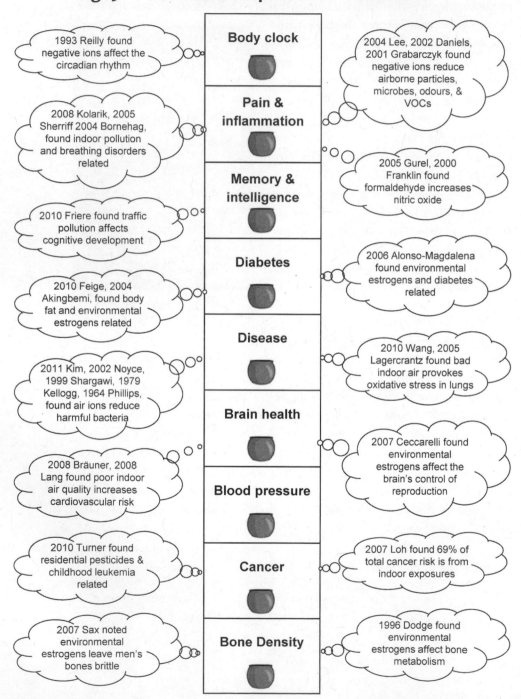

1993 Reilly found negative ions affect the circadian rhythm

2004 Lee, 2002 Daniels, 2001 Grabarczyk found negative ions reduce airborne particles, microbes, odours, & VOCs

2008 Kolarik, 2005 Sherriff 2004 Bornehag, found indoor pollution and breathing disorders related

2005 Gurel, 2000 Franklin found formaldehyde increases nitric oxide

2010 Friere found traffic pollution affects cognitive development

2006 Alonso-Magdalena found environmental estrogens and diabetes related

2010 Feige, 2004 Akingbemi, found body fat and environmental estrogens related

2011 Kim, 2002 Noyce, 1999 Shargawi, 1979 Kellogg, 1964 Phillips, found air ions reduce harmful bacteria

2010 Wang, 2005 Lagercrantz found bad indoor air provokes oxidative stress in lungs

2008 Bräuner, 2008 Lang found poor indoor air quality increases cardiovascular risk

2007 Ceccarelli found environmental estrogens affect the brain's control of reproduction

2010 Turner found residential pesticides & childhood leukemia related

2007 Loh found 69% of total cancer risk is from indoor exposures

2007 Sax noted environmental estrogens leave men's bones brittle

1996 Dodge found environmental estrogens affect bone metabolism

Body clock

Pain & inflammation

Memory & intelligence

Diabetes

Disease

Brain health

Blood pressure

Cancer

Bone Density

Dilute

Outdoor air can be used to dilute the high levels of pollutants in some homes, although there are homes located near busy roads, freshly sprayed golf courses, and in more polluted cities where that may not be such a great idea. In areas with good air, simply open the windows for ten minutes before going to bed, after taking baths and showers, after cooking, and after hobby activities.

Reduce

In homes where the windows really can't be opened, it becomes even more important to keep the sources of indoor pollutants to a minimum.

Mold can usually be contained by dealing with the moist, nutrient-rich conditions where it's likely to make an appearance. Clean humidifier trays and air conditioners. Be sure to maintain areas where moisture from outside is likely to gain entry — around downspouts and roof guttering. If a small mold farm does appear, it can usually be cleaned up by moistening, wiping, moistening again, scrubbing with a brush and wiping the area clean. Some dishwashing detergents, like Palmolive, are particularly effective against mold.

Larger mold farms may need to be dealt with professionally. As long as the source of moisture has been removed, increasing the ventilation to the area should prevent the mold from becoming re-established.

Radon remediation is usually done by professionals and involves trapping and venting the gases from the affected area to the top of the building where it can be carried away by air currents.

Chemicals can be reduced by limiting the number of personal care, cleaning and fragranced products in use, storing them in a separate air space, keeping bathroom doors closed, and relocating computers and entertainment, hobby setups and storage areas away from the bedroom.

Many of the chemicals that come into bedrooms enter from new carpets, furnishings and ensuite bathrooms. Airing out carpets and furniture before bringing it into the bedroom reduces these chemicals – it can take as long as six months. Adding a resin-charcoal base to water softeners removes chlorine from your water, reducing the amount that enters the bedroom from ensuite bathrooms. Shower units that

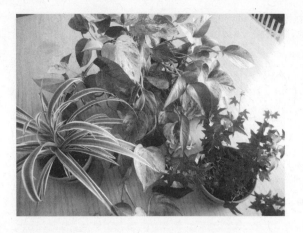

Clay pots and foliage add charge neutral surfaces and remove some chemicals from the air

Photo:
Angela Hobbs

dechlorinate the water during a shower are available, but charcoal tends to be more effective with cold water.

Plants can be very effective at reducing the chemicals in your air, although some scientists think they're overrated.[11] It takes several plants to noticeably reduce the chemicals in a 100ft^2 room. Some like pothos, Boston ferns, spider plants, Areca palms, ivy, and peace lilies are better known for their air-cleaning qualities. Unhealthy plants can add ethylene,[12] to your air and should be removed. Soils that have been kept wet enough for mold growth, or treated with insecticides recently, should be kept out of the bedroom.

Barricade

Windows, doors, seals, and diversions, all help to prevent pollutants from entering the bedroom. Closing bathroom doors and windows usually keeps any off-gassing from personal care products, traffic and garden treatments out of the bedroom.

Carefully positioned ventilation inlets and radon pipes can prevent unwanted air pollutants from the ground, neighbouring dryers and heating/cooling outlets from entering your home.

Sealing lids of products that smell and sealing connections to attached garages and chimneys keeps air pollutants from leaking into the house.

Increasing air ions

Minimizing synthetic surfaces and maximize charge-neutral surfaces leaves more ions in the air. Ideally, the square footage of natural surfaces should be greater than that of synthetic ones (or at least the same). Charge-neutral surfaces are naturally occurring and include wood, cotton, natural linoleum, bamboo, vegetable fibre, sisal, coir, and sea grass. Several items in the typical bedroom are available in natural materials, including bedding, bed skirts, window treatments, wall hangings, tablecloths, throws, stuffed toys, storage containers and furniture.

Air ions can also be increase by using unglazed clay pots for healthy plants, opening the windows and/or running a cold shower for five minutes before turning in for the night.

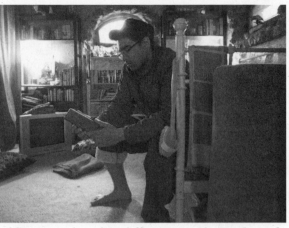

An air ion meter eliminates Sandeep's radon concerns. To fix his ion depleted air he needs less stuff, more natural surfaces and fresh air

Photo:
Angela Hobbs

It's not unusual for bedrooms to be cleaned last — after all no-one is going to see them. But dusting and vacuuming weekly can make a big difference to the quality of the air you breathe through the night.

Summary

Studies have shown that when particulate levels rise, a rat's blood thickens and slows and its nitric oxide levels shoot up by 350 percent, damaging the lining of its blood vessels and lungs.[13] (I'm sure I'm not alone in thinking that's a good thing: more airborne particulates = fewer rats.) Unfortunately, the argument extends to humans, too. Rising air pollution outdoors correlates with increased deaths from asthma, pneumonia, emphysema, heart attacks, and strokes.[14] Efforts to increase the energy efficiency of our homes have had a disastrous effect on their air quality. Some estimates suggest that the air in the average home is about five times more polluted than outdoor air, while others feel that estimate is far too conservative.

With every move toward energy efficiency, every installation of synthetic fabrics and furnishings, every occurrence of personal care products and cleaners, and every move to use the bedroom space for more than just sleep, the air in our bedrooms becomes more polluted. Bad air in the bedroom rapidly translates into poor sleep and ill health. More pollutants arrive with every new synthetic surface, and with every new synthetic surface there are even fewer ions left in the air to rid it of pollutants and prevent them gaining direct access to the lungs.

While we may not be able to influence the level of air pollution outside, the levels in our bedrooms are eminently controllable. Limiting the synthetic materials and products that gain access to the bedroom and replacing furnishings with natural unfinished products that won't deplete the air's ion content are good starting points. The improved air in the room where we spend about a third of our lives pays dividends in sleep quality and overall health and sets the immune system up to take the day's hostilities in its stride.

Part 3 — How to Power Up Your Sleep

9 — Putting It All Together

A self-help program for better bedrooms

Until now we've looked at noise, microwaves, light, electricity, contact chemicals, and air pollutants in isolation. But they don't often occur in isolation; they usually occur in combinations that build on each other to provoke the sleep/wake conflict. Recognizing them and knowing which one to tackle first is a common conundrum – where do you start?. In this chapter, we'll meet Mia and we'll work through her situation. You'll see how we identified the culprits, how she set about dealing with them, and the difference that understanding her bedroom environment made to her life. We'll end with a "how-to" guide and a worksheet so that you too can transform your bedroom to one that's more conducive to sleep and health.

Mia's Story

Mia and her family had moved from Norway to downtown Kelowna, British Columbia when her husband transferred jobs. They'd bought a house in what seemed like a quiet residential neighbourhood, but after a few months she and her family were exhausted and having a hard time adjusting to their new home.

Several times every night, Mia, her husband, and their two children would be woken by the sirens of ambulances, fire trucks, or police cars. Annoyed, they would try to settle back in their beds, only to be awoken again by the next emergency vehicle. After six months, they were all sharing a windowless room in the basement.

Mia explained to me that in Norway, legislation and public awareness was focused on promoting quiet. Even small noises were targeted. She was dismayed to find that in Kelowna, the law stated that emergency vehicles

133

had to put their sirens on whenever they deviated from the rules of the road, even in the dead of night. She wished with all her heart that they hadn't bought this house in what was clearly the wrong neighbourhood.

"I don't know what to do," she told me. "My husband is always angry, my children hate their school, and I'm so tired all the time that I can't remember a thing or get anything done."

Although the noise from the emergency vehicles was the most obvious sleep impediment that Mia and her family were dealing with, and the one she'd asked for help with, it turned out to be far from the only one.

Assessing Mia's Master Bedroom

Noise

The noise from the emergency vehicle sirens was by far the most significant source of noise at night, but there was also some road noise from passing vehicles that didn't have sirens. Other sources included the window air conditioner, the dripping tap in the ensuite bathroom, and the ticking and cuckooing of the cuckoo clock.

Microwaves

There were several sources of microwaves in Mia's house in addition to the cell phone tower two blocks away. Her cordless phone, wireless doorbell, wireless internet router, the children's Wii, and the security system were all making a significant contribution to the ease with which the family was awakened through the night.

Light

The lightweight window coverings that had come with the house were doing little to keep out the streetlight. But there were also other light sources in the bedroom: a radio alarm with a large blue display, a computer monitor with a rotating screen saver, a white night light in the hallway, and a lighted electronic picture frame with revolving pictures.

Electricity

The radio alarm, computer, cell phone chargers, and electronic picture frame, along with the transformers that converted the household AC to their DC power were all creating EMFs in the bedroom. The air conditioner in the window was an obvious source; less obvious was the old, inefficient fridge in the kitchen below (remember, EMFs travel through walls, floors, and ceilings). The metal coils in the couple's spring mattress were ensuring that all these EMFs were captured and kept right next to their bodies through the night.

Contact Chemicals

Although Mia and her husband used cotton bedding, the old washing machine that came with the house wasn't doing a great job of rinsing out the detergent, so Mia had resorted to a fragranced fabric softener to take the stiffness out of the fabric. The whole family slept in polyester pajamas.

Air Pollutants

Although the couple used a cotton duvet cover and a wooden bureau to store their clothes, most of the surfaces in their bedroom were synthetic, including the carpet, washable walls, night stands, and reclining chair. In addition to this, there were no doors on either the ensuite bathroom or the walk-in closet, and that meant the chemicals from a whole host of toiletries and dry cleaning had direct access to their air. Because they used the master bedroom as a quiet space to catch up on correspondence, it also housed the computer and printer.

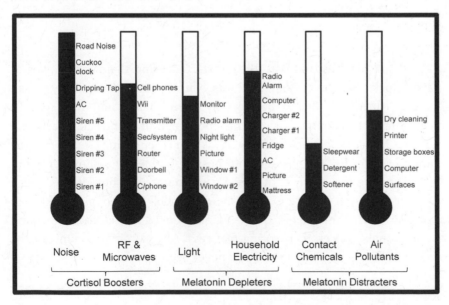

Mia's Master Bedroom

When she was finished recording the things she could improve on, Mia's meter looked like this

What Mia Did to the Master Bedroom

Once we'd filled in the Mistake Meter for the master bedroom, Mia was able to prioritize her approach to transforming her bedroom. As would be expected in her situation, the tallest column was noise, so she started here. With that column reduced she went on to the next tallest column — household electricity. Then she went on to deal with the next tallest column, microwaves, followed by light and air pollutants, before turning her attention to her shortest column, which was contact chemicals.

Noise

The first thing Mia did was to fill any holes and cracks under the trim around the windows. Next she added storm windows with an inner sound-absorbent pad around the frame, to all the windows. She replaced the lightweight curtains with heavier sound-absorbent ones. Mia and her husband removed the window air conditioner so that they could get a good seal on this window, too. If all their efforts made the house livable, they would invest in central air conditioning before the heat of the summer set in. The couple also fixed the dripping tap in the ensuite bathroom, put a couple of panel absorbers in the corners of each of the bedrooms to reduce the hum of the traffic, and removed the battery from the cuckoo clock. From now on it would be a quiet ornament.

Electricity

Mia and her husband had already started using their cell phones as alarm clocks, so the radio alarm was simply thrown out. They began charging their cell phones before they went to bed and replaced the electronic picture frame with a conventional frame and their favourite picture. Mia created an "activity nook" in the dining room for the computer and its peripherals and began unplugging equipment and gadgets before the family turned in for the night. The old kitchen fridge was replaced with a more efficient newer model. The couple decided to wait and see if the changes they'd made reduced the electricity around them enough to keep their spring mattress. After all, it had come all the way from Norway with them and had never been a problem in the past.

Microwaves

Mia and her husband were terribly curious about the microwaves. They hadn't even noticed the cell phone tower, and had never lived in homes that didn't come equipped with a cordless phone, wireless doorbell, wireless internet router, and wireless security system. To see the signals that were hitting the family's pillows we used a spectrum analyzer. The couple was stunned to actually "see" something invisible. In response they quickly painted the wall facing the cell tower with conductive Y-shield paint and grounded it. At night they made sure they turned off the children's remote-controlled toys and Wii, and they replaced their wireless systems with wired ones. Now that they were conscious of the microwaves, they began setting their cell phones to airplane mode at night – that way they'd work as alarm clocks without transmitting through the night. Once the new normal was established, we used the spectrum analyzer again to identify areas where the microwave signals were fewest and weakest and moved the head of the beds into one of these areas.

Light

By the time Mia got to this column, she had already dealt with many of the problems. The heavier curtains had reduced the light penetrating the windows from the street lights; the radio alarm with its large blue display had been thrown out; the computer was down in the dining room; and the lighted electronic picture frame had been replaced with a stationary, unlit picture of the children. What remained was the white night light in the hallway, and that was simply replaced with a red bulb.

Air Pollutants

The first thing the couple did to reduce this column was install doors on the ensuite bathroom and walk-in closet. They threw out the toiletries they were no longer using and aired their dry cleaning before hanging it in the closet. With the computer and printer already moved to the activity nook in the dining room, and heavy cotton curtains adorning the windows, most of the issues in this column had already been dealt with. But they saw an opportunity to increase the natural surfaces in their bedroom even more by replacing their particleboard night stands with wooden ones, hanging some large bamboo feng shui art work on the walls, and bringing in a couple of air-cleaning plants. The reclining chair found a new home in the living room, and Mia replaced the old washing machine with its pathetic rinse with one that had an additional rinse cycle. That quickly eliminated any need for a fabric softener.

Contact Chemicals

The new washing machine took care of the detergent residues, so that when Mia got to this column the remaining opportunity for improvement was to replace the family's polyester sleepwear with cotton.

Assessing the Children's Bedroom

By the time Mia had transformed her own bedroom, many of the issues that had initially affected the children's room had been dealt with. We used the list on page 144 to help identify exposures and prioritize the challenges in the children's room.

Noise

With all the sound in the house no one had noticed just how noisy the fish tank was. Now its humming aerator and trickling water stood out.

Microwaves

The Wii and remote-controlled cars were both microwave sources in this bedroom.

Light

The white light in the fish tank, the flimsy curtains that allowed the street light to flood the room, and the white night light made this a very bright bedroom.

Electricity

Both of the children slept on space-saving metal bunk beds – the type with a raised bed that allows room for a desk below the sleeper. One of the children was sleeping above a computer and printer plugged into a surge protector. The other was sleeping above an electric keyboard with its transformer plugged into a surge protector. The fish tank aerator was also plugged into a surge protector, along with a battery charger and several other AC/DC transformers that charged the children's toys.

Contact Chemicals

Most evenings the children took showers before they went to bed in their polyester pajamas. Their beds were made up with polyester bedding on foam mattresses.

Air Pollutants

The children's bedroom seemed to almost double as a playroom, which meant there were several sources of air pollutants in it. Like most playrooms, it was full of plastic storage boxes and washable surfaces. There was also a computer, electric keyboard, hobby supplies, and an open laundry hamper filled to the brim with what smelled like damp towels and dirty socks. One of the walls had clearly suffered from a moisture problem caused by a broken roof gutter, but although the gutter had been fixed, the moisture issues that it had created in the wall remained — the moldy smell in the room couldn't all be blamed on the laundry hamper, and couldn't be disguised by the air freshener. There were absolutely no natural surfaces in this bedroom.

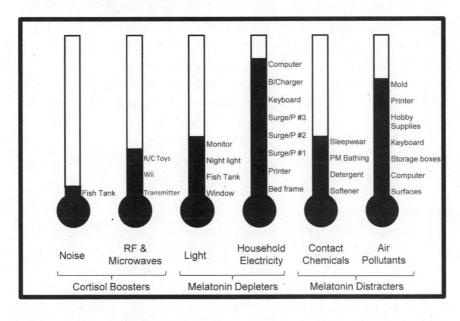

Mia's Children's Bedroom

When the assessment was finished the children's meter looked like this

What Mia did in the Children's Bedroom

The tallest columns in this room were electricity and air pollutants, followed by the light, contact chemicals, microwaves, and the noise being created by the fish tank. As she had done in the master bedroom Mia tackled the children's room beginning with the tallest column and working her way down to the shortest.

Electricity

The computer, printer, electric piano, and hobby supplies moved down into new "activity nooks" in the living room and den. Two of the surge protectors went with them, to be unplugged at night, while the third one was put away. The children learned to unplug their chargers when they weren't using them, and the fish tank found a new home in the living room. Since the metal bunk beds were brand new, the family decided to hold on to them for a while.

Air Pollutants

Tackling the mold issue in the children's bedroom turned out to be a little more work than Mia and her husband had bargained for. Once they ripped out the drywall, they discovered a fully-grown mold farm all over the wood and insulation. The whole wall had to be gutted, cleaned and rebuilt before they could tackle any of the other issues.

Once that was done, Mia went to work replacing some of the synthetic surfaces with natural ones that would improve the room's ion content. She started by removing the air freshener, replacing the plastic storage containers with wicker baskets, and switching the polyester bedding for cotton. The laundry hamper got a lid and she made sure to watch for wet towels going into it. Moving the computer, printer, electric piano and hobby supplies had helped address this column, too.

Contact Chemicals

The children were thrilled with their new cotton duvet covers and now Mia tackled the rest of the bedding. She covered their foam mattresses with thick cotton bedspreads and replaced their polyester pajamas with cotton ones. Her new washing machine with its extra rinse cycle meant she no longer relied on her fabric softener to soften the children's clothes and bedding. She also insisted that the children start taking their baths and showers on weekends or in the morning before school.

Light

Mia hung heavy cotton curtains on the windows and replaced the white bulb in the children's night light with a red one.

Microwaves

By now most of the microwave sources in the home had been dealt with, and as long as someone remembered to unplug the Wii and take the batteries out of the remote-controlled cars, there was little else to do. As we'd done in the master bedroom, we used the spectrum analyzer to identify areas where any microwaves entering the room from outside were weakest and fewest and then moved the heads of the children's beds into these areas.

Now that Mia understood more about microwaves and how they keep the awake system going, ultimately shortening the night, she made an effort to change the family's routine. She began encouraging the children to turn off their equipment earlier in the evening and enjoying quiet, low-stress chats with them during the hour before they went to bed.

Noise

Since the siren noise coming through the windows had been dealt with and the fish tank had moved downstairs, the bedroom now had no noise issues to deal with.

Before long, Mia's husband was less quick to anger, while the children began adjusting to their school and making some new friends. Mia began sleeping well and felt better able to cope with her new life away from the supports of family and friends. She signed up for a course and discovered she could volunteer in the children's school. Soon she was getting to know some of the other mothers. Mia's future, and that of her growing family, began looking as bright as it had when they'd agreed to her husband's transfer.

Do It Yourself

Like Mia, and many others, you can use the approach outlined below to identify the things in your bedroom that may be contributing to your sleepless nights and ill health. As with Mia, there are probably restrictions on what you can achieve. Maybe a family member insists on operating particular equipment through the night, or maybe you live on a noisy street. It could be the proximity of a cell phone transmitter, or a neighbour's wind turbine, even motorbikes being revved up at 2 a.m. Remember, the goal here isn't to achieve perfection, but rather to be supportive to the normal hormonal flow — to prevent any unnecessary sleep/wake conflict.

Identifying mistakes is usually far more of a challenge than fixing them. Complications may come as you try to decide which group a mistake belongs in. **It doesn't matter**. The real point is that the more groups it belongs in, the more reasons you have to get rid of it.

1. Armed with a pen, a blank meter and list on pages 144 and 145, go into the bedroom.

2. Use the list to help you figure out what you're looking for. Look for:

    -   **Noise** – any sound that regularly leaps out of the background at night.

    -   **Microwaves** – any transmitter closer to your pillow than 7 metres (approx 20 feet) unless otherwise specified in the chart. It's present on a regular basis at night. Microwaves travel through walls, floors, and ceilings, so the sources of concern won't necessarily be in the bedroom.

    -   **Light** – any light (other than moonlight, starlight and red light) that allows you to see shadows once you've settled for the night. You should not be able to read with the lights out.

    -   **Electricity** – any electrical outlet, wiring, appliance or gadget (and any battery-powered gadget) closer to your head during sleep than 2 metres (six feet) unless otherwise specified in the chart. It's present on a regular basis at night. Like microwaves, electromagnetic fields travel through walls, floors, and ceilings, so the sources of concern won't necessarily be in the bedroom.

    -   **Contact chemicals** – any synthetic, chemically-treated, or chemical-containing product that comes into contact with your skin on a regular basis at night.

    -   **Air pollutants** – any synthetic surface, container, or fan-equipped appliance that contributes chemicals or depletes ions on a regular basis at night.

3. As you identify sources of each of these elements, record them in the appropriate column.

- Some of them, like an air conditioner, TV, or fan, will qualify for more than one column. Record it wherever you want to, multiple times if you like. The more columns it fits in, the more reasons you have to get it out of the bedroom.
- Some of them will be hidden from view — the sockets behind the headboard, the plastic shoe storage under the bed, the air freshener under the laundry pile. Hidden or obvious, write it down.

4. Once your meter's complete, pick the tallest column and ask yourself:

- Which of these sources am I going to fix?
- How am I going to deal it? What works with my budget and my situation?
- Can I move it out of the bedroom?
- Can I turn it off at night?
- Can I increase the distance?
- Can I compensate?

5. Revisit the chapter that deals with the source you're considering; it should give you some ideas to try.

- Noise page 37
- Microwaves page 53
- Light page 69
- Electricity page 79
- Contact chemicals page 97
- Air pollutants page 111

6. If you deal with a source that you've recorded in more than one column, remove it from all of the columns.

7. When you've implemented the fixes you are able to make for the tallest column, start on the next tallest column and run through steps 1-6 again.

Common Sleep Disruptors

Noise	Microwaves	Light	Magnetic Fields	Chemicals	Air Pollutants
Air conditioner	Airport radar (<1km)	Bathroom light	Major power line or substation (<1km)	Bedtime bathing	Ailing plants
Airplanes	Cell phone mast (<300m)	Bright outside lights	Distribution line or transformer (<15m)	Body lotion	Air freshener
Barking dog	Baby monitor	Clock radio display	Air conditioner/ purifier/humidifier	Detergent residues	Busy road, or gas station (<50m)
Busy road					
Ceiling fan	Cell phone	Curtainless window	Baseboard heater	Fabric softeners	Ceiling fan
Cuckoo clock	Computer peripherals	Fish tank light	Battery clock Bedside lamp	Fabric treatments	Cleaning products
Dishwasher	Cordless phone	Fluorescent light	CO/smoke detector	Foam mattress	Cleaning residues
Dripping tap	Doorbell	LED displays	Ceiling fan	Moisturizer	Computer
Fish tank air supply	GPS	Neighbour's lights	Computer & peripherals	Perfumes	Detergent residues
Fridge	Internet PlayStation peripherals	Reading light	Electric blanket	Personal care products	Dry cleaning
Heat pump					
Humming lights	Remote car starter	Street lights	Electric panel	Polyester bedding	Fabric treatments
Leaky windows	Remote-controlled toys	White night light	Electric sockets	Polyester bra	Flea collars
Mice			Garage door opener		Foam mattress
Music	Satellite navigation system		Inverter	Polyester pillow	Hobby supplies
Noisy neighbours	Security system		Major appliances	Polyester sleepwear	Laundry basket
Pets			Metal bed frame		Incense/candle
Radio/TV	Scanner		Radio	Shampoo	Mold/odour
Sirens	Smart meter		Recharger/transformer	Soap	Personal care products
Snoring partner	TV/radio mast (<1km)		Shaver, toothbrush	Wrinkle releasers	Plastic storage boxes
Ticking clocks	Wii peripherals		Solar panels (<3m)		Printer inks
Trains			Stetzer Filters		Storage
Ventilation system			Surge protector		Stuffed toys
Water softener			Timers		Synthetic surfaces
Wind farm (<2km)			TV/DVD/stereo		TV

Mistake Meter Work Sheet

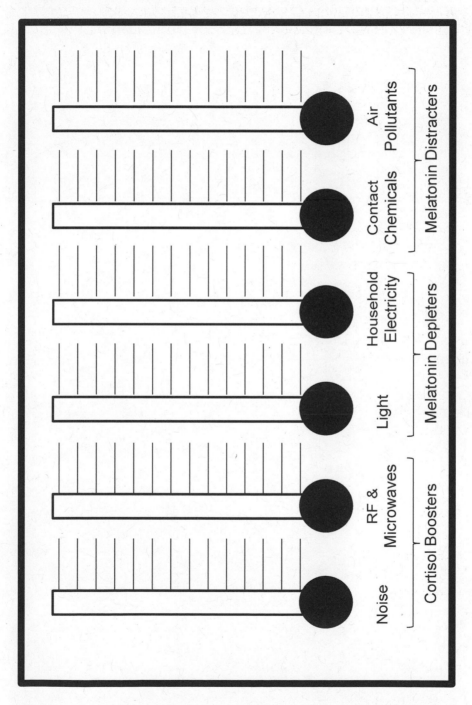

10 — Daytime Is Playtime — If Night's Right!

What's next?

The last century saw more changes to our living environment than at any other time in history, and the speed of that change has had consequences. Changing our surroundings faster than we can adapt to them has given rise to new conditions, new illnesses, and new diseases.

With those changes, though, have come greater knowledge, understanding, and communication. We know more about the human body, more about communicating, more about disease, and a great deal more about sleep than we did a century ago. But while much has been accomplished, much remains to be done, because all those accomplishments aren't yet being channelled toward the one thing that makes them all worthwhile and sustainable — our health. What we have to do now is pool the knowledge available to us from other cultures, other countries, other times and other ways, and use it to create the twenty-first century toolkit that will allow us to navigate health and buy us the time to adapt to all the changes we've made and those yet to come.

Media-enabled Change

The pace of change through the last century was greatly facilitated by the common belief in technology as a solution and by the growing reach of the media, especially television. This new equipment that brought moving pictures right into our living rooms reached the masses in a way that nothing else had. It transcended literacy boundaries, established a broadly shared vision of the future, and paved the way for new products.

Until these broadcasts arrived in our homes, any vision of the future was limited to those who were interested and literate enough to seek it out, those with access to Buck Rogers newspaper cartoons, Isaac Asimov's *Foundation Trilogy*, or Jules Verne's *Twenty Thousand Leagues Under The Sea*. With the new equipment poised right in the middle of the living room, even the most disinterested and illiterate were almost guaranteed to catch at least a glimpse of the future embodied in Gene Roddenberry's *Star Trek* and Glen Larson's *Battlestar Galactica*.

Our growing familiarity with this compelling and achievable future paved the way for new products. It made us comfortable with "communicators" that flipped open and with the wireless network they connected to. It made us comfortable with shiny washable surfaces. It made us comfortable with tight-fitting, easy-care clothing. It made us comfortable with ergonomically designed work stations — preferably with molded, swivelling chairs and a whole lot of buttons to push. It made us comfortable with boxes that beeped to announce our speedily cooked food was ready to eat. When those products arrived in our stores, we were ready for them. We greeted every advance toward our shared vision of the future with open arms. No description of these cool new toys ever came with a cautionary tale.

While television paved the way for the rapid influx of products, it missed the mark in three areas that would eventually become critical. It didn't reveal the health impact that would inevitably accompany the rapid changes to our indoor environment. It usually presented society's enemies as alien creatures, complete with arms and legs. And it depicted the great outdoors as a vast dark space full of twinkling stars, big enough to swallow anything we might want to throw at it.

Entrepreneurs Turn to Less Regulated Opportunities Indoors

The dramatic pace of change indoors was greatly helped along by events transpiring outside. The ecology movement, with Rachel Carson at the helm, was steadily reigning in the unfettered innovation and research that was harming the great outdoors. In *Silent Spring,* Carson alerted the world to the crazy situation she'd uncovered. Governments were supporting the massive spraying of DDT, even though no one could explain how it killed insects and no one had considered the impact that the absence of those insects would have on the rest of the food chain. Carson left us with a warning to "reach beyond our grasp" — to recognize that if something provokes a response in dose quantities, overdosing can have far-reaching consequences.

Entrepreneurs and researchers now turned their attention to innovations for use indoors, where less attention was being paid to safety and the standards were more lax. Products could — and were, and continue to be — brought to the market with minimal testing, on the assumption that people won't buy something that can harm them. Regulations based on the concept of self-effacing products greatly reduced the time it took to bring a product to market. Unfortunately the public assumed those products wouldn't be permitted for sale if they were harmful!

Our Desensitized Alarm Levels

Had the self-effacing concept been followed through to its logical conclusion, a product would have to be taken off the shelves when it hurt someone — at least until more was understood about how it hurt them and safeguards could be put in place. But instead of blaming dangerous products or ingredients, we began labeling the people who were hurt by these products...and kept the products on the market. As we ignored and medicated our human "canaries," our hurt consumers appeared in droves — they were asthmatic, allergic, chemically sensitive, and electrically sensitive. They had insomnia, vibrational sensitivities, attention deficits, learning disabilities, memory impairments, migraines, diabetes, heart and pain conditions, and so on. Unaware that they were canaries, they accepted their diagnosis and expressed their gratitude for whatever chemicals the pharmaceutical industry could offer to ease their suffering and mask their symptoms. Most don't even suspect that the products they've brought into their homes might be related to the sleep issues and ill health they've succumbed to.

Today those "sensitivities" and "illnesses" are well established and our willingness to dismiss the dangers posed by products that should have been "self effacing" is complete. That leaves a vast horizon for the clever entrepreneur — someone who's not necessarily trying to hurt anyone, but who's focused on corporate growth. These are people who know how to read the market, who see product gaps years before the rest of us even glimpse them, who persuade us of our need for their product long before it's launched, and who are masters at creating a demand.

Misplaced trust in manufacturers and a sense of complacency have endangered our health. As a result all that equipment and all those products have introduced sleep disrupters into our homes. We've become so accustomed to receiving a constant signal bombardment from noise, microwaves, odors, light, and electricity that we don't even notice we're desensitized. To provoke us into action, signals have to reach critical intensities — our smoke detectors have to screech, gas leaks and poor sanitation odors have to be overwhelming, and lights have to flash brighter, faster, and longer to get our attention. By being unaware of low-level signals we are left vulnerable to disease, a vulnerability we amplify by tricking our bodies into sleep rather than listening to them and adjusting the signals they interpret as warnings.

Without proper sleep, there can be little pleasure in the products we bring into our lives. To be able to enjoy today's conveniences, efficiencies, and luxuries in the daytime, we have to know when to stop using them at night. Ultimately, daytime is a more enjoyable, energetic, and invigorating playtime when we sleep properly.

Reaching Beyond Our Grasp - Indoors

If we were to really "reach beyond our grasp," and put our health first we would need a more strongly regulated environment "indoors". One that: delivered internet signals through existing electrical systems (distributed by fiber-optic not wireless); located electric panels, solar panels and inverters away from bedrooms; banned smart meters, community internet, and CFL light bulbs; insisted bedroom furniture be made from unfinished wood; encouraged the use of plastic-free, charge-neutral, paints in bedrooms; eliminated synthetic bedding materials; declared homes built over distortions in the Earth's magnetic fields uninhabitable; and moved the brickwork so often found outside our homes inside where it could increase the ion count. Maybe we could even subsidize Dyson vacuum cleaners.

For most of us modifying our entire homes to this extent is simply too much, but the bedroom as a small, contained area where we spend several healing hours at a time, is an ideal place to start.

What's Next?

One of the main contributions to poor sleep is the absence of conversation that surrounds it. Typically when someone shows signs of, or comments on, not having slept well, they're avoided. No one wants to deal with a grouch and no one really knows what to suggest.

That conversation avoidance results in utter misery for a good third of the population anticipating yet another night of sleep deprivation, and another day of fatigue and sheer exhaustion. It affects their relationship not just with you, but with their co-workers, their families, and their communities. It affects their productivity, their confidence, their creativity, and their interest in the world around them.

Occasionally a sleep-deprived person will decide to try something to improve their sleep: a new sleep medication, a yoga class, or changing some nuance of sleep hygiene. Or they may have developed a suspicion that there's something in the bedroom and want to try a different room. More often than not, the minute she voices her idea, it's met with ridicule: "Oh, she's just fixated on the loud cars that leave the pub at three in the morning," or "If you stopped focusing on it, you'd have a better perspective," or "If I was worrying about sleeping this much, I wouldn't be able to sleep either."

If instead of raising a sleep issue the person commented about food or exercise, we'd all have something to suggest. If they commented about persistent indigestion or their weight gain, we'd be able to suggest a variety of diets, if they revealed concern about their lack of exercise; we'd know what to say. That conversational willingness that surrounds diet and exercise issues encourages people to keep looking for answers, to keep talking, to keep asking questions. **But** conversation avoidance about sleep issues breeds ridicule and ultimately isolation and desperation — poor sleepers end up having to seek medical intervention for something they used to do just fine. Before you know it they'll have a diagnosis, one that will quickly become their identity, and once that happens the opportunity to alert them to the possible contribution that their bedroom is making will be lost forever.

You'll provoke some very interesting, helpful conversations by leaving this book lying around! Those conversations will relieve the isolation and desperation that someone in your midst is experiencing right now. When your friends, family and co-workers see the book, they'll start asking the questions they should be asking. A question says, "I'm ready to hear this." Leaving it on the coffee table will start your family and friends thinking about the distance that their bedroom has come from the "sleep well, feel well" conditions created in those holiday places they love to escape to. And once they start thinking about it, they'll start doing some of the little things that can make such a huge difference to their sleep and health.

Ultimately, they'll begin to understand that being equipped to live healthily in the twenty-first century takes more than a good diet and ample exercise. In this new world, "daytime is playtime," but only if "night's right."

References

Introduction

[1] Boffetta, P., "Fruit and vegetable intake and overall cancer risk in the European prospective investigation into cancer & nutrition (EPIC)." *J. Natl. Cancer Inst.*, Vol. 102 (8), 2010, p 529-537

[2] Gregory, J.M., "Sleep management for farm families." *Healthy Farmer*, Vol. 3, 2007.

[3] Boyd, D.R. and S.J. Genuis. "The environmental burden of disease in Canada: respiratory disease, cardiovascular disease, cancer, & congenital affliction". *Environmental Research*, Vol. 106 (2), 2008, p. 240-249

Chapter 1 — Sleep Isn't Optional

[1] Gregory, J.M., "Sleep management for farm families." *Healthy Farmer*, Vol. 3, 2007.

[2] Williams, R., *The Trusting Heart: Great News about Type A Behaviour.* Crown, 1989

[3] Barchas, J.D., "Aaron Lerner: Perspectives & lessons learned from the melatonin days." *J. Investigative Dermatology*, Vol. 127, 2007 p. 2085-2089

[4] Lerner, A.B. et al., "Isolation of melatonin, a pineal factor that lightens melanocytes." *J. American Chemical Society*, Vol. 80, 1958, p. 2587

[5] Selye, H., *The Stress of My Life; A Scientist's Memoirs.* Van Nostrand Reinhold, 1979

[6] Reiter, R.J., [online] *"Melatonin and its Metabolites."* [accessed September 2009] http://sciencewatch.com/inter/pod/a2/ January 2008

[7] Foster, R.G. and L. Kreitzman, *Rhythms of life: the biological clocks that control the daily lives of every living thing.* Yale University Press. 2004

[8] Tolan, T., [online] *"Rico visits Erling Andechs & the Max Planck Bunker."* [accessed Feb. 2009] www.stanfordalumni.org/travelswithrico/54BunkerTalk.htm

[9] Jurgen Aschoff Obituary. *Current Science*, Vol. 75 (12), 1998 [accessed Mar. 2009] www.ias.ac.in/jarch/currsci/75/00001440.pdf

[10] Vijayalaxmi et al., "Melatonin as a radioprotective agent: a review." *Int. J. Radiation Oncology, Biology, Physics*, Vol. 59 (3), 2004 p. 639-653

[11] Griefahn, B. et al., "Autonomic arousals related to traffic noise during sleep." *Sleep*, Vol. 31 (4), 2008, p. 569-577

[12] Aeschbach, D. et al., "A longer biological night in long sleepers than short sleepers." *J. Clin. Endocrinology & Metab.*, Vol. 88 (1), 2003, p. 26-30.

Bass J., "Sleepless In America : A pathway to obesity and the metabolic syndrome?" *Archives of Internal Medicine*, Vol. 165, 2005, p. 15-16

Blask, D.E., "Melatonin as a chronobiotic/anticancer agent: cellular, biochemical & molecular mechanisms of action & their implications for circadian based cancer therapy." *Curr. Top. Med. Chem.*, Vol.2, 2002, p.113-132

Bonnet, M.H. and D.L. Arand, "Hyperarousal & insomnia: state of the science." *Sleep Medicine Reviews*, 2010. Vol. 14 (1) p. 9-15

Crabtree V.M. et al., "Periodic limb movement disorder of sleep in children." *J. Sleep Research*, Vol. 12, 2003, p. 73-81

Dexter, J. D. and T. L. Riley, "Studies in nocturnal migraine." *Headache*, Vol. 15, 1975, p. 51-62

Dimitrov, S. et al., "Sleep associated regulation of T helper 1/T helper 2 cytokine balance in humans." *Brain, Behav. Immun.*, Vol.18, 2004, p.341-48.

Elwood, P. et al., "Sleep disturbance, stroke, and heart disease events: evidence from the Caerphilly Cohort." *JECH*, Vol. 60 (1), 2006, p.69-73

Fogel, S. M. and C. T. Smith, "Learning-dependent changes in sleep spindles and stage 2 sleep." *J. Sleep Research*, Vol. 15 (3), 2006, p. 250–255

Foley D, et al., "Sleep disturbances & chronic disease in older adults." *National Sleep Foundation Sleep in America Survey*, 2003

Gottlieb D.J. et al., "Symptoms of sleep-disordered breathing in 5-year-old children are associated with sleepiness & problem behaviors." *Pediatrics*, Vol. 112, 2003, p. 870–877

Kang J., "Amyloid-Beta dynamics are regulated by orexin & the sleep-wake cycle." *Science*, Vol. 326, 2009, p. 1005-1007

Killgore W.D.S. et al., "Sleep deprivation reduces perceived emotional intelligence & constructive thinking skills." *Sleep Medicine*, Vol. 9 (5), 2008, p. 517–526

Knutson, K.K.L. et al., "Association between sleep & blood pressure in midlife: the CARDIA sleep study." *Archives of Internal Medicine*, Vol. 169 (11), 2009, p. 1055–1061

Knutsson, A., "Health disorders of shift workers." *Occ. Med.*, Vol. 53 (2), 2003, p.103–108

Elwood, P. et al., "Sleep disturbance, stroke, & heart disease events: evidence from the Caerphilly Cohort." *JECH*, Vol. 60 (1), 2006, p. 69–73

Levi F. et al., "Circadian timing in cancer treatments." *Annual Review of Pharmacology & Toxicology*, Vol. 50, 2010, p. 377-421

Lopes, M.C. et al., "Delta sleep instability in children with chronic arthritis." *Brazilian J. Med. & Biological Res.*, Vol. 41 (10), 2008, p. 938–943.

Miller, M.A. and F.P. Cappuccio, "Inflammation, sleep, obesity & cardiovascular disease." *Current Vascular Pharm.*, Vol. 5, 2007, p. 93–102

Moldofsky, H., "Pain & insomnia: what every clinician should know." *Medscape Neurology & Neurosurgery*, Vol. 6 (2), 2004.

Paavonen, E.J. et al., "Short sleep duration and behavioral symptoms of attention-deficit/hyperactivity disorder in healthy 7-8 year-old children." *Pediatrics*, Vol. 123 (5), 2009, p. 857–864

Schwartz, W.J., "Understanding circadian clocks: from c-Fos to fly balls." *Annals of Neurology*, Vol. 41 (3), 1997, p. 289–297

Sephton S. and Spiegel D., "Circadian disruption in cancer: a neuroendocrine-immune pathway from stress to disease?" *Brain, Behavior, & Immunity*, Vol. 17 (5), 2003, p. 321-328

Spiegel, K. et al., "Impact of sleep debt on physiological rhythms." *Revue Neurologique*, Vol. 159 (S.11), 2003, p. 11–20

Spiegel, K. et al., "Sleep curtailment in healthy young men is associated with decreased leptin levels, elevated ghrelin levels, & increased hunger & appetite." *Annals of Internal Medicine*, Vol. 141 (11), 2004, p. 846–850

Van Cauter, E. et al., "The impact of sleep deprivation on hormones & metabolism." *Hormone Research*, Vol. 67 (S.1), 2007, p. 2–9

Vgontzas, A.N. et al., "Selective effects of CPAP on sleep apnoea-associated manifestations." *Eur. J. Clin. Invest., Vol. 38 (8), 2008, p. 585–595*

[13] Roth, T., "Comorbid insomnia: current directions & future challenges." *Am. J. Manag. Care,* 2009. Vol. 15 (S), p. 6-13

Chapter 2 — How Disrupted Sleep Impacts Your Health

[1] Lavie, P., "Sleep-wake as a biological rhythm." *Annual Review of Psychology*. Vol. 52, 2001, p. 277–303.

Pandi-Perumal, S.R. et al., "Role of the melatonin system in the control of sleep: therapeutic implications." *CNS Drugs*, Vol. 21 (12), 2007, p. 995–1018.

[2] Ishida A, et al., "Light activates the adrenal gland: timing of gene expression & glucocorticoid release." *Cell Met.*, Vol. 2 (5), 2005, p. 297–307

[3] Navara, K.J. and Nelson, R.J., "The dark side of light at night: physiological, epidemiological & ecological consequences." J. *Pineal Res.*, Vol. 43, 2007, p.215–24

[4] Claustrat, B. et al., "The basic physiology and pathophysiology of melatonin." *Sleep Medicine Reviews*, Vol. 9 (1), 2005, p. 11–24

[5] Heymfield, S. B., "Recombinant leptin for weight loss in obese & lean adults." *JAMA*, Vol. 282 (16), 1999, p. 1568–1575

[6] Spiegel, K., "Sleep curtailment in healthy young men is associated with decreased leptin, elevated ghrelin, & increased hunger & appetite." *Ann. Intern. Med.*, Vol. 141, 2004, p. 846–850

[7] Gangwisch, J.E. et al., "Sleep duration as a risk factor for diabetes incidence in a large U.S. sample." *Sleep*, Vol. 30 (12), 2007, p. 1667–1673

[8] Miller, M.A. and P.F., Cappuccio. "Inflammation, sleep, obesity & cardiovascular disease." *Curr. Vasc. Pharmacology*, Vol. 5, 2007, p. 93–102

[9] Cutolo, M. et al., "Circadian rhythms: glucocorticoids & arthritis. *Ann. New York Academy of Sciences*, Vol. 1069 (1), 2006, p. 289–299

[10] De Weerth, C. et al., "Development of cortisol circadian rhythm in infancy." *Early Human Development*, Vol. 73 (1-2), 2003, p. 39–52

Pandi-Perumal, S.R. et al., "Role of the melatonin system in the control of sleep: therapeutic implications." *CNS Drugs*, Vol. 21, 2007, p. 995–1018

[11] Van Cauter, E. et al., "The impact of sleep deprivation on hormones & metabolism." *Hormone Research*, Vol. 67 (S1), 2007, p. 2–9

[12] Reiter, R.J. et al., "When melatonin gets on your nerves: its beneficial actions on experimental models of stroke." *Experimental Biology & Medicine*, Vol. 230 (2), 2005, p. 104–117

[13] Coyle, J.T. and P. Puttfarcken, "Oxidative stress, glutamate & neurodegenerative disorders." *Science*, Vol. 262, 1993, p. 689–95

Granot, E. and R. Kohen, "Oxidative stress in childhood health & disease states." *Clinical Nutrition*, Vol. 23 (1), 2004, p. 3–11

Schulz, J.B. et al., "Glutathione, oxidative stress & neurodegeneration." *European J. Biochemistry*, Vol. 267 (16), 2000, p. 4904–4911

[14] Zeman M. et al., "Plasma melatonin concentrations in hypertensive patients with the dipping & non-dipping blood pressure profile." *Life Sciences*, Vol. 76, 2005, p. 1795–1803

Tengattini, S., "Cardiovascular diseases: protective effects of melatonin." *J. Pineal Research*, Vol. 44, 2008, p.16–25

Ohkubo T., et al., "Relation between nocturnal decline in blood pressure & mortality: the Ohasama Study." *American J. Hypertension*, Vol. 10, 1997, p. 1201–1207

Muller J.E. et al., "Circadian variation & triggers of onset of acute cardiovascular disease." *Circulation*, Vol. 79, 1989, p. 733-743

Stergiou G.S. et al., "Parallel morning & evening surge in stroke onset, blood pressure, & physical activity." *Stroke*, Vol. 33, 2002, p. 1480–1486

Brugger P. et al., "Impaired nocturnal secretion of melatonin in coronary heart disease." *The Lancet,* Vol. 345, 1995

[15] Jacks, B., "Melatonin." *Alive Magazine,* July 2007.

[16] Korkmaz, A. et al., "Role of melatonin in the epigenetic regulation of breast cancer." *Breast Cancer Research & Treatment,* Vol. 115, 2009, p. 13–27

[17] Park, S.Y. et al., "Melatonin suppresses tumor angiogenesis by inhibiting HIF-1alpha stabilization under hypoxia." *J. Pineal Research,* Vol. 48, 2010, p. 178–184

[18] Leon-Blanco, M.M. et al., "Melatonin inhibits telomerase activity in the MCF-7 tumor cell line both in vivo & in vitro." *J. Pineal Research,* Vol. 35 (3), 2003, p. 204–211

Hacket, J.A. and C.W. Greider, "Balancing instability: dual roles for telomerase & telomere dysfunction in tumorigenesis." *Oncogene,* Vol. 21, 2002, p. 619–626

Hug, N and J. Lingner, "Telomere length homeostasis." *Chromosoma,* Vol. 115 (6), 2006, p. 413-25

Lung, F.W. et al., "Genetic pathway of major depressive disorder in shortening telomeric length." *Psychiatric Genetics,* Vol. 17, 2007, p. 195–199

Harst, P. et al. "Telomere length of circulating leukocytes is decreased in patients with chronic heart failure." *J. American College of Cardiology,* Vol. 49, 2007, p. 1459–1464

Fitzpatrick, A.L. et al., "Leukocyte telomere length and cardiovascular disease in the cardiovascular health study." *American J. Epidemiology,* Vol. 165, 2007, p. 14–21

Cawthon, R.M. et al., "Association between telomere length in blood & mortality in people aged 60 years or older." *The Lancet,* Vol. 361, 2003, p. 393–395

Kimura, M. et al., "Telomere length & mortality: a study of leukocytes in elderly Danish twins." *Am. J. Epidemiology,* Vol. 167, 2008, p. 799–806

[19] Serra V, et al., "Extracellular SOD is a major antioxidant in human fibroblasts & slows telomere shortening." *J. Biological Chemistry,* Vol. 278, 2003, p. 6824–6830

[20] Sanchez-Hidalgo, M. et al., "Melatonin inhibits fatty acid-induced triglyceride accumulation in ROS17/2.8 cells: implications for osteoblast differentiation & osteoporosis." *American J. Physiology,* Vol. 292 (6), 2007, p. 2208–2215

[21] Shultz, T.D. et al., "Decreased intestinal calcium absorption in vivo & normal brush border membrane vesicle calcium uptake in cortisol-treated chickens: evidence for dissociation of calcium absorption from brush border vesicle uptake." *Proc. Natl. Acad. Sci.* Vol. 79 (11), 1982, p. 3542–3546

[22] Alesci, S. et al., "Glucocorticoid-induced osteoporosis: from basic mechanisms to clinical aspects." *Neuroimmunomodulation,* Vol. 12 (1), 2005, p. 1–19

Birketvedt, G.S. et al., "HPA axis in the night eating syndrome." *Am. J. Physiol. Endocrinol. Metab,* Vol. 282 (2), 2002, p. 366–369

Born J. and H. Fehm, "The neuroendocrine recovery function of sleep." *Noise & Health,* Vol. 2 (7), 2000, p. 25–38

Cos, S. et al., "Estrogen-signalling pathway: a link between breast cancer & melatonin's oncostatic actions." *Cancer Detect. Prev.,* Vol. 30 (2), 2006, p. 118–128

Cutando, A. et al., "Melatonin: potential functions in the oral cavity." *J. Periodontology,* Vol. 78 (6), 2007, p. 1094–1102

Ekstedt M, et al., "Arousals during sleep are associated with increased levels of lipids, cortisol & blood pressure." *Psychosom. Med.,* Vol. 66, 2004. p. 925–931

Elenkov, I.J. and G.P. Chrousos, "Stress hormones, proinflammatory & antiinflammatory cytokines, & autoimmunity." *Ann. N.Y. Acad. Sci.,* Vol. 966, 2002, p. 290–303

Epel E.S. et al., "Dynamics of telomerase activity in response to acute psychological stress." *Brain, Behavior, & Immunity*, Vol. 24, 2010, p. 31-39

Gorfine, T. et al., "Sleep-anticipating effects of melatonin in the human brain." *Neuroimage*, Vol. 31 (1), 2006, p. 410–418

Gutierrez-Cuesta, J. et al. "Chronic administration of melatonin reduces cerebral injury biomarkers in SAMP8." *J. Pineal Research*, Vol. 42 (4), 2007, p. 394–402

Lavie, P., "Melatonin: role in gating nocturnal rise in sleep propensity." *J. Biological Rhythms*, Vol. 12 (6), 1997, p. 657–665

Leon-Blanco, M.M. et al., "Melatonin inhibits telomerase activity in the mcf-7 tumor cell line both in vivo & in vitro." *J. Pineal Research*, Vol. 35, 2003, p. 204–211

Mead, M. and M. Nathaniel, "The sound behind heart effects." *EHP*, Vol. 115 (11), 2007, p. 536–537

Paulis, L. et al., "Minireview, Blood pressure modulation & cardiovascular protection by melatonin: potential mechanisms behind." *Physiological Research*, Vol. 56, 2007, p. 671–684

Pena, C. et al., "Chemotactic effect of melatonin on leukocytes." *J. Pineal Research*, Vol. 43 (3), 2007, p. 263–269

Quiros, I. et al., "Melatonin prevents glucocorticoid inhibition of cell proliferation & toxicity in hippocampal cells by reducing glucocorticoid receptor nuclear translocation." *J. Steroid Biochem. Mol. Biol.*, Vol. 110 (1-2), 2008, p. 116–124

Reiter, R.J., "Oxygen radical detoxification processes during aging: the functional importance of melatonin." *Aging*, Vol. 7 (5), 1995, p. 340–51

Saarela, S. and R.J. Reiter, "Function of melatonin in thermoregulatory processes." *Life Sciences*, Vol.54 (5), 1994, p. 295–311

Sainz, R. M. et al., "Melatonin regulates glucocorticoid receptor: an answer to its antiapoptotic action on thymus." *Federation of American Societies for Experimental Biology*, Vol. 13 (12), 1999, p. 1547–1556

Saretzki, G. and T. von Zglinicki, "Replicative aging, telomeres, & oxidative stress." *Ann. New York Academy of Sciences*, Vol. 959, 2002, p. 24–29

Torres-Farfan, C. et al., "MT1 melatonin receptor in the primate adrenal gland: inhibition of adrenocorticotropin-stimulated cortisol production by melatonin. *J. Clinical Endocrinology & Metabolism*, Vol. 88 (1), 2003, p. 450–458

Takechi, M, et al. "Effect of FGF-2 & melatonin on implant bone healing: a histomorphometric study." *JMSMM* , Vol. 19 (8), 2008, p. 2949–2952

Vgontzas, A.N. and G.P. Chrousos, "Sleep, the HPA axis, & cytokines: multiple interactions & disturbances in sleep disorders." *Endocrinology & Metabolism Clinics of North America*, Vol. 31 (1), 2002, p. 15–36

Chapter 3 — Noise and Infrasound

[1] Evans, G.W. et al., "Chronic noise exposure & physiological response: a prospective study of children living under environmental stress." *Psychological Science*, Vol. 9, 1998, p. 75–77

[2] Stansfeld, S. A. et al., "Aircraft & road traffic noise & children's cognition & health: a cross-national study." *The Lancet*, Vol. 365, 2005, p. 1942–1949

[3] Siegel, J. M., "Why we sleep." *Scientific American*, Vol. 289 (5), 2003, p. 92–97

[4] Alves-Pereira M. et al., "Vibroacoustic disease: biological effects of infrasound & low-frequency noise explained by mechanotransduction cellular signalling." *Progress in Biophysics & Molecular Biology*, Vol. 93 (1–3), 2007, p. 256–279

[5] WHO, [online] Night Noise Guidelines for Europe, 2009. [accessed Jan 2011] http://www.euro.who.int/document/e92845.pdf

[6] Hughes, D., The Energy Issue: A more Urgent Issue than Climate Change. In Homer-Dixon, T. *Carbon Shift: How the Twin Crises of Oil Depletion and Climate Change Will Define the Future.* Random House Canada, 2009

[7] Sean Whittaker, VP Policy Canadian Wind Energy Association, interview with Anna Maria Tremonti "Against the Wind," CBC Radio, 2009

[8] Anna Maria Tremonti, "Against the Wind," CBC Radio, 2009

[9] Berglund, B. et al., [Online] "Guidelines for Community Noise." WHO (1999). Cited Jan. 2009 http://whqlibdoc.who.int/hq/1999/a68672.pdf

[10] Ministry of the Environment, Ontario (2009). "Wind turbines - proposed requirements & setbacks". [Accessed Jun. 2010] http://news.ontario.ca/ene/en/2009/06/backgrounder-wind-turbines---proposed-requirements-and-setbacks.html

[11] ISO International Standards Organization 2631 (2003)

[12] Rasmussen, G., "Human body vibration exposure & its measurement", *J. Acoustical Society of America,* Vol. 73 (6) 1983, p. 2229

[13] Frey, B.J. et al., [online] "Noise radiation from wind turbines installed near homes: effects on health." FRICS 2007. [accessed Mar. 2009] www.windturbinenoisehealthhumanrights.com

[14] Babisch, W. and I. van Kamp, "Exposure-response relationship of the association between aircraft noise & the risk of hypertension." *Noise & Health,* Vol. 11 (44), 2009, p. 161–8

Babisch, W. et al., "Blood pressure of 8-14 year old children in relation to traffic noise at home: results of the German environmental survey for children." *Science of the Total Environment,* Vol. 407, 2009, p. 5839–5843

Basner, M. et al., "Effects of nocturnal aircraft noise." *Deutsches Zentrum fur Luft und Raumfahrt,* Bericht 2004-07/E

Berglund, B. et al., "Sources & effects of low Noise." *J. the Acoustical Society of America,* Vol. 99, 1996, p. 2985–3002

Bluhm G. et al., "Road traffic noise & annoyance: an increasing environmental health problem." *Noise & Health.* Vol. 6 (24), 2004, p. 43–9

Carter, N.L., "Transportation noise, sleep, & possible after-effects." *Environment International,* Vol. 22. 1996. p. 105–116

Danielsson, Å. and U. Landström, "Blood pressure changes in man during infrasonic exposure: an experimental study." *Acta Medica Scandinavica,* Vol. 217 (5), 1985, p. 531–535

De Boer, S.F. et al., "Adaptation of plasma catecholamine & corticosterone responses to short-term repeated noise stress in rats." *Physiology & Behavior,* Vol. 44 (2), 1988, p. 273–280

Griefahn B. and Spreng M., "Disturbed sleep patterns & limitation of noise." *Noise & Health,* Vol. 6 (22), 2004, p. 27-33

Haralabidis, A. et al., "Acute effects of nighttime noise exposure on blood pressure in populations living near airports." *European Heart Journal,* Vol. 29 (5), 2008, p. 658–664

Ising, H. and M. Ising, "Chronic cortisol increases in the first half of the night caused by road traffic noise." *Noise & Health,* Vol. 4, 2002, p. 13–21

Ising H. et al., "Respiratory & dermatological diseases in children with long-term exposure to road traffic emissions." *Noise & Health,* Vol. 5 (19), 2003, p. 41–50

Ising, H. et al., "Low frequency noise & stress: bronchitis & cortisol in children exposed chronically to traffic noise and exhaust fumes." *Noise & Health,* Vol. 6 (23), 2004, p. 21–28

Jarup, L. et al., "Hypertension & exposure to noise near Airports: the HYENA study." *EHP*, Vol. 116 (3), 2008, p. 329–33

Maschke, C. and K. Hecht, "Stress hormones & sleep disturbances: electrophysiological & hormonal aspects." *Noise & Health*, Vol. 6 (22), 2004, p. 49–54

Manikandan S. et al., "Antioxidant property of alpha-asarone against noise-stress-induced changes in different regions of rat brain." *Pharmacol. Res.*, Vol. 52 (6), 2005, p. 467–474

McCarthy, D.O., "Shades of Florence Nightingale: potential impact of noise stress on wound healing." *Holist. Nurs. Practice*, Vol. 5, 1991, p. 39–48

Ravindran R. et al., "Noise-stress-induced brain neurotransmitter changes & the effect of Ocimum sanctum (linn) treatment in albino rats." *J. Pharmacol. Sci.*, Vol. 98, 2005, p. 354–360

Selander, J. et al., "Saliva cortisol & exposure to aircraft noise in six European countries." *EHP*, Vol. 117 (11), 2009, p. 1713–1717

Spreng, M., "Noise induced nocturnal cortisol secretion & tolerable overhead flights." *Noise & Health*, Vol. 6 (22), 2004, p. 35–47

van Kempen E.E. et al., "Children's annoyance reactions to aircraft & road traffic noise." *J. Acoust. Soc. Am.*, Vol. 125 (2), 2009, p. 895–904

Verzini, A.M. et al., "A field research about effects of low frequency noises on man." *Acta Acustica*, Vol. 85, 1999, p. 16

Visser, O. et al., "Incidence of cancer in the area around Amsterdam Airport Schiphol in 1988–2003: A population-based ecological study." *BMC Public Health*, Vol. 5, 2005, p. 127

Waye, K.P. et al., "Cortisol response & subjective sleep disturbance after low-frequency noise exposure." *J. Sound & Vibration*, Vol. 277 (3), 2004, p. 453–457. Fifth Japanese-Swedish Noise Symposium on Medical Effects.

WHO, [online] Night Noise Guidelines for Europe, 2009. [accessed Jan. 2010] http://www.euro.who.int/document/e92845.pdf

Wysocki A.B. "The effect of intermittent noise exposure on wound healing." *Advances In Wound Care*, Vol. 9 (1), 1996, p 35–39

Chapter 4 — Radio Frequency and Micro Waves

[1] Lilienfeld, A.M. et al., "Evaluation of health status of foreign service & other employees from selected eastern European embassies." final report; Contract No. 6025-619037 (NTIS publication P8-288 163/9) 1978

[2] Dalton L., *Radiation Exposures*, Scribe Publications, p. 31, 1991

[3] Maisch, D. [Online] *The Procrustean Approach; Setting Exposure Standards for Telecommunications Frequency Electromagnetic Radiation*, Ph.D. Thesis, 2010. http://www.iemfa.org/images/pdf/The_Procrustean_Approach.pdf

[4] Sakharchuk, I.I. et al., "The use of MRT in peptic ulcer with concomitant liver involvement." *Vrachebnoe Delo*, 1990, p. 83–85

Dziublik, A.A. et al., "The use of MRT on patients with chronic nonspecific lung diseases." *Vrachebnoe Delo*, 1989, p. 55–56

Efimov, A.S. et al., "The effect of MRT on the clinical & metabolic indices of diabetic patients." *Ter. Arkhiv*, Vol. 63 (10), 1991, p. 51–54

Puryshkina, O.D., "Microwave Resonance Therapy in the combined treatment of eczema." *Likars'ka sprava*, 1999, p. 94–97

Jovanović-Ignjatić, Z. and D. Raković, "A review of current research in MRT: novel opportunities in medical treatment." *Acupuncture & Electro-Therapeutics Research*, Vol. 24 (2), 1999, 105–125

5 Santini, R. et al., "Study of the health of people living on the vicinity of mobile phone base stations: influence of distance & sex." *Electromagn. Biol. Med.*, Vol. 22 (1), 2003, p. 41–49

6 Vom Saal, F., *BPA References.* [accessed Jan. 2010] http://endocrinedisruptors.missouri.edu/vomsaal/vomsaal.html

7 Abdel-Rassoul, "Neurobehavioral effects among inhabitants around mobile phone base stations." *Neurotoxicology*, Vol. 28, 2007, p. 434–440

Altpeter, E. S. et al., "Effect of short-wave (6-22 MHz) magnetic fields on sleep quality & melatonin cycle in humans: the Schwarzenburg shut-down study." *Bioelectromagnetics*, Vol. 27 (2), 2006, p. 142–150

Blank, M. and R. Goodman, "EMFs stress living cells." *Pathophysiol., Vol.* 16, 2009, p. 71–78

Bortkiewicz, A. and P. Medycyna, "A study on the biological effects of exposure mobile-phone frequency EMF." *Med. Pr.*, Vol. 52, 2001, p. 101–106

Boscol, P. et al., "Effects of EMF produced by radiotelevision broadcasting stations on the immune system of women." *Sci. Total Environ.*, Vol. 273 (1-3), 2001, p. 1–10

Chiang, H. et al., "Health effects of environmental electromagnetic fields." *J. Bioelectricity*, Vol. 8, 1989, p.127–131

Dolk, H. et al., "Cancer incidence near radio & television transmitters in Great Britain." *American J. Epidemiology*, Vol. 145 (1), 1997, p. 1–9

Eger, H. et al., [online] "The influence of being physically near to a cell phone transmission mast on the incidence of cancer." *Umwelt Medizin Gesellschaft*, Vol. 17 (4), 2004. [accessed Jul. 2010] www.tetrawatch.net/papers/naila.pdf

Fesenko, E. E. et al., "Microwaves & cellular immunity. Effect of whole body microwave irradiation on tumor necrosis factor production in mouse cells." *Bioelectrochemistry & Bioenergetics*, 49 (1), 1999, p. 29–35

Ha, M., et al., "RF radiation exposure from am radio transmitters & childhood leukemia & brain cancer." *American J. Epidemiology*, Vol. 166 (3), 2007, p. 270–279

Hocking, B. et al., "Cancer incidence, mortality & proximity to TV towers." *Medical J. Australia*, Vol. 165 (11-12), 1996, p. 601–605

Huber R. et al., "EMFs, such as those from mobile phones alter regional cerebral blood flow & sleep & waking EEG." *J. Sleep Research*, Vol. 1 (4), 2002, p. 289–295

Hutter, H. P. et al., "Subjective symptoms, sleeping problems, & cognitive performance in subjects living near mobile phone base stations." *Occupational & Environmental Medicine.* Vol. 63 (5), 2006, p. 307–313

Lai H, et al., "Naltrexone blocked RFR-induced DNA double strand breaks in rat brain cells." *Wireless Networks Journal*, Vol. 3, 1997 p. 471–476

Li, M. et al., "Elevation of plasma corticosterone levels & hippocampal glucocorticoid receptor translocation in rats: a potential mechanism for cognition impairment following chronic low-power-density microwave exposure." *J. Radiation Research*, Vol. 49 (2), 2008, p. 163–70

Lotz, W.G. and R.P. Podgorski, "Temperature & adrenocortical responses in rhesus monkeys exposed to microwaves." *J. Appl. Physiol.*, Vol. 53 (6), 1982, p. 1565–1571

Lu, S.T. et al., "Delineating acute neuroendocrine responses in microwave-exposed rats." *J. Applied Physiology*, Vol. 48, 1980, p. 927–932

Mann, et al., "Effects of pulsed high-frequency EMFs on the neuroendocrine system." *Neuroendocrinology*, Vol. 67, 1998, p. 139–144

Michelozzi, P. et al., "Adult & childhood leukemia near a high-power radio station in Rome, Italy." *Am. J. Epidemiol.*, Vol. 155, 2002, p. 1096–1103

Nittby, H. et al., "Cognitive impairment in rats after long-term exposure to GSM-900 mobile phone radiation." *Bioelectromagnetics*, Vol. 29 (3), 2008, p. 219–232

Novoselova, E.G. et al., "Microwaves & cellular immunity. immunostimulating effects of microwaves & naturally occurring antioxidant nutrients." *Bioelectrochem. Bioenerg.*, Vol. 49 (1), 1999, p. 37–41

Oberfeld, G. et al., [Online] "The microwave syndrome-further aspects of a Spanish study." *Conference Proceedings*, Kos Greece, October 2004. [accessed Oct. 2010] www.powerwatch.org.uk/pdfs/20040809_kos.pdf

Panagopoulos, D. J. et al., "Bioeffects of mobile telephony radiation in relation to its intensity or distance from the antenna." *Int. J. Rad. Biol.*, Vol. 86, 2010, p. 345–57

Pérez-Castejón, C. et al., "Exposure to ELF-pulse modulated x band microwaves increases in vitro human astrocytoma cell proliferation." *Histology & Histopathology*, Vol. 24, 2009, p. 1551–156

Persson, B.R.R. et al., "Blood-brain barrier permeability in rats exposed to EMFs used in wireless communication." *Wireless Network*, Vol.3, 1997, p. 455–461

REFLEX Consortium (2004) Final Report. [accessed Apr. 2010] www.Verum-Foundation.De/Reflex

Sabanayagam, C. and A, Shankar, "Sleep duration & cardiovascular disease: results from the national health interview survey." *Sleep*, Vol. 33 (8), 2010

Salama, N. et al., "Effects of exposure to a mobile phone on testicular function and structure in adult rabbit. *Int. J. Androl*, Vol. 33, 2010, p. 88–94

Santini, R. et al., "Study of the health of people living in the vicinity of mobile phone base stations: influence of distance and sex." *Electromagn. Biol. Med.*, Vol. 22 (1), 2003, p. 41–49

Sinha, R.K., "Chronic non-thermal exposure of modulated 2450 MHz microwave radiation alters thyroid hormones & behavior of male rats." *Int. J. Radiat. Biol.*, Vol. 84, 2008, p.505–513

Stankiewicz, W. et al., "Immunotropic influence of 900 MHz microwave GSM signal on human blood immune cells activated in vitro." *Electromagn. Biol. Med.*, Vol. 25, 2006, p. 45–51

Szmigielski, S. et al., "Alteration of diurnal rhythms of blood pressure & heart rate to workers exposed to radiofrequency EMFs." *Blood Pressure Monitoring*, Vol. 3 (6), 1998, p. 323–330

Vangelova, K. et al., "The effect of low level radiofrequency electromagnetic radiation on the excretion rates of stress hormones in operators during 24-hour shifts." *Central European J. Public Health*, Vol. 10 (1- 2), 2002, p. 24–28

Vangelova, K. et al., "Changes in excretion rates of stress hormones in medical staff exposed to electromagnetic radiation." *Environmentalist*. Vol. 227, 2007, p. 551–555

Yariktas, M. et al., "Nitric Oxide level in the nasal and sinus mucosa after exposure to EMF." *Archives of Otolaryngology — Head & Neck Surgery*, Vol. 132 (5), 2005, p. 7136

Yurekli, A.I., et al., "GSM base station electromagnetic radiation and oxidative stress in rats." *Electromagn. Biol. Med.*, Vol. 25, 2006, p. 177–188

Wolf, D. and & D. Wolf. "Increase of cancer near cell-phone transmitter station." *International J. Cancer Prevention*, Vol. 1–2, 2004

[8] Johnson, D., [online] *Better Together, How cooperation could cut energy wastage in the UK mobile phone industry*. 2009 [accessed Jan 2010], http://leamington.greenparty.org.uk/assets/files/reports/Better_Together.pdf)

Chapter 5 — Light

[1] Murray, L. et al., "The cognitive development of 5-year-old children of postnatally depressed mothers." *J. Child Psychology & Psychiatry*, Vol. 37 (8), 1996, p. 927–35

[2] Lockley, S.W. et al., "High sensitivity of the human circadian melatonin rhythm to resetting by short wavelength Light." *J. Clin. Endocrinol. Metab.*, Vol. 88 (9), 2003, p. 4502–4205

[3] Baade, P.D., "International epidemiology of prostate cancer: geographical distribution and secular trends." *Molecular Nutrition & Food Research*, Vol. 53 (2), 2009. p. 171–184

[4] IARC Press Release No. 180

[5] Davidson, A. J. et al., "Chronic jet-lag increases mortality in aged mice." *Current Biology*, Vol. 16, 2006, p. 914–916

[6] Ben-Shlomo, R, and C.P. Kyriacou, "Light pulses administered during the circadian dark phase alter expression of cell cycle associated transcripts in mouse brain." *Cancer Genetics & Cytogenetics*, Vol. 197 (1), 2010, p. 65–70.

Blask, D. E., "Growth & fatty acid metabolism of human breast cancer (mcf-7) xenografts in nude rats: impact of constant light-induced nocturnal melatonin suppression." *Breast Cancer Research & Treatment*, Vol. 79 (3), 2003, p. 313–320

Blask D.E. et al., "Melatonin-depleted blood from premenopausal women exposed to light at night stimulates growth of human breast cancer xenografts in nude rats." *Cancer Research*. Vol. 65, 2005, p. 11174-11184

Brainard, G.C. et al., "Action spectrum for melatonin regulation in humans: evidence for a novel circadian photoreceptor." *J. Neuroscience*, Vol. 21 (16), 2001, p. 6405–6412

Cajochen C, et al., "High sensitivity of human melatonin, alertness, thermoregulation, & heart rate to short wavelength light." *J. Clin. Endocrinol. Metab.*, Vol. 90 (3), 2005, p. 1311–1316

Davidson, A.J. et al., "Block chronic jet lag increases mortality in aged mice." *Current Biology*, Vol. 16, 2006, p. 914–916

Duffy, J.F., et al., "Entrainment of the human circadian system by light." *J. Biological Rhythms*, Vol. 20 (4), 2005, p. 326–338

Haines V.Y. et al., "The mediating role of work-to-family conflict in the relationship between shiftwork & depression." *Work Stress*. Vol. 22, 2008, p.341–56

Hansen J., "Light at night, shiftwork & breast cancer risk." *J. National Cancer Institute*, Vol. 93, 2001, p. 1513–1515

Ishida A, et al., "Light activates the adrenal gland: timing of gene expression & glucocorticoid release." *Cell Metab.*, Vol. 2, 2005, p. 297–307

Kloog, I. et al., "Light at night co-distributes with incident breast but not lung cancer in the female population of Israel." *Chronobiol. Int.*, Vol. 25, 2008, p. 6–8

Knutsson, A. and H. Bøggild, "Shift work, risk factors & cardiovascular disease." *Scand. J. Work, Environment & Health*. Vol. 25 (2), 1999, p. 85-99

Kristensen, T.S., "Cardiovascular diseases & the work environment: a critical review of the epidemiologic literature on nonchemical factors." *Scandinavian J. Work, Environment & Health*. Vol. 15, 1989, p. 165-179

Kyriacou, C. P. et al., "Circadian clocks: genes, sleep, and cognition." *Trends in Cognitive Sciences*. Vol. 14 (6), 2010, p. 259-267

162

Lavie, P., "Sleep-wake as a biological rhythm." *Annu. Rev. Psychol.*, Vol. 52, 2001, p. 277–303

Lewy, A. J., "Circadian misalignment in mood disturbances." *Current Psychiatry Reports,* Vol. 11 (6). 2009, p. 459-465

Ostrowska, Z. et al., "Influence of lighting conditions on daily rhythm of bone metabolism in rats & possible involvement of melatonin & other hormones in this process," *Endocrine Regulations*, Vol. 37, 2003, p. 163–174

Pandi-Perumal, S.R. et al., "Role of the melatonin system in the control of sleep." *CNS Drugs,* Vol. 21 (12), 2007, p. 995–1018

Pukkala, E. et al., "Does incidence of breast cancer and prostate cancer decrease with increasing degree of visual impairment." *Cancer Causes & Control,* Vol. 17 (4), 2006, p. 573–576

Srinivasan, V. et al., "Therapeutic actions of melatonin in cancer: possible mechanisms." *Int. Cancer Therapies,* Vol. 7 (3), 2008, p. 189–203

Stevens, R.G., "Artificial lighting in the industrial world: circadian rhythm disruption & breast cancer risk." *Cancer Causes & Control,* Vol. 17, 2006, p. 501–507

Suwazono, Y. et al., "Longitudinal study on the relationship between alternating shift work and the onset of diabetes mellitus in Japanese workers." *J. Occup. Environ. Med.,* Vol. 48, 2006, p. 455–461

Thapan, K, et al., "An action spectrum for melatonin suppression: evidence for a novel non-rod, non-cone photoreceptor system in humans." *J. Physiology,* Vol. 535 (1), 2001, p. 261–267

Tokura H. et al., "Effects of bright and dim light intensities during daytime upon circadian rhythm of core temperature in man." In Milton, A.S. (ed.) *Temperature Regulation.* Birkhäuser Verlag, Basel, 1994, p. 285–289

Trinder, J. et al., "Inhibition of melatonin secretion onset by low levels of illumination. *J. Sleep Research,* Vol. 5 (2), 1996, p. 77–82

Chapter 6 — Household Electricity and the Earth's Magnetic Fields

[1] Fagan, B., *From Black Land to Fifth Sun: The Science of Sacred Sites.* Addison-Wesley, 1998

[2] Resch, J., "Geographic distribution of multiple sclerosis & comparison with geophysical values". *Soz Praventivmed*, Vol. 40 (3), 1995, p. 161-171.

[3] Warren, S. et al., "Incidence of Multiple Sclerosis among First Nations People in Alberta, Canada." *Neuroepidemiology*, Vol. 28 (1), 2007, p. 21–27

[4] Svenson, L.W. et al. "Prevalence of Multiple Sclerosis in First Nations People of Alberta." *Can. J. Neurol. Sciences,* Vol. 34 (2), 2007, p. 175 – 180

Svenson, L.W. et al., "Regional variations in the prevalence rates of Multiple Sclerosis in the province of Alberta, Canada." *Neuroepidemiology.* Vol. 13 (1-2), 1994,p. 8-13

Pugliatti, M. et al., "The epidemiology of Multiple Sclerosis in Europe." *European J. Neurology.* Vol. 13, 2006, p. 700–702

Atlas Multiple Sclerosis resources in the world 2008. WHO [online] http://www.who.int/mental_health/neurology/Atlas_MS_WEB.pdf p. 14

Cheng, Q. et al., "Multiple Sclerosis in China--history and future." *Multiple Sclerosis,* Vol. 15 (6), 2009, p. 655-660.

[5] Persinger, M.A., "A potential multiple resonance mechanism by which weak magnetic fields affect molecules & medical problems: the example of melatonin & experimental 'Multiple Sclerosis." *Medical Hypotheses,* Vol. 66 (4), 2006, p. 811–815

Martin, T.D. et al., "Mood effects of prefrontal repetitive high-frequency TMS in healthy volunteers." *CNS Spectrums*, Vol. 2, 1997, p. 53

Klein, E. et al., "Therapeutic efficacy of right prefrontal slow repetitive TMS in major depression." *Archives of General Psychiatry*, Vol. 56 (4), 1999, p. 315–320

Elahi, B. et al., "Effect of TMS on Parkinson motor function--systematic review of controlled clinical trials." *Movement Disorders*, Vol. 24 (3), 2009, p. 357–363

Centonze D, et al., "Repetitive TMS of the motor cortex ameliorates spasticity in Multiple Sclerosis." *Neurology*, Vol. 68 (13), 2007, p. 1045–1050

Clarke, B. M. et al., "TMS for migraine: clinical effects." *J. Headache Pain*, Vol. 7 (5), 2006, p. 341–346

[6] Von Pohl, G.F., *Earth Currents, Causative Factor of Cancer and other Diseases*, Frech-Verlag, Germany 1988

[7] Hartmann, E., *Illness as a Problem of Location.*, Karl F. Haug Verlag, Germany 1964

[8] Wertheimer, N. and E. Leeper, "Electric wiring configurations & childhood cancer." *International J. Epidemiology*, Vol. 109, 1979, p.273–284

[9] Feychting, M. and A. Ahlbom, "Magnetic fields & cancer in children residing near Swedish high-voltage power lines." *American J. Epidemiology*, Vol. 138, 1993, p. 467–481

[10] Linet, M. S. et al., "Residential exposure to magnetic fields & acute lymphoblastic leukemia in children." *NEJM*, Vol. 337, 1997, p. 1–7

[11] Milham, S. and E.M. Ossiander, "Historical evidence that residential electrification caused the emergence of the childhood leukemia peak." *Med. Hypotheses*, Vol. 56, 2001, p. 290–295

[12] Ahlbom, A. et al., "A pooled analysis of magnetic fields & childhood leukaemia." *British J. Cancer.* Vol. 83 (5), 2000, p. 692-698.

Blank, M. and R. Goodman, "EMFs stress living cells." *Pathophysiology*, Vol. 16, 2009, p.71-78

Brendel, H, et al., "Direct suppressive effects of weak magnetic fields (50 Hz and 16 2/3 Hz) on melatonin synthesis in the pineal gland of Djungarian hamsters." *J. Pineal Research*, Vol. 29 (4), 2000, p. 228-233

Burch J. B. et al., "Geomagnetic activity and human melatonin metabolite excretion." *Neuroscience Letters*, Vol. 438 (1), 2008, p. 76-79

Cansevan, A., "Suppression of natural killer cell activity on Candida stellatoidea by a 50Hz magnetic field." *J. Cell Biochemistry.* Vol. 99 (1), 2006, p. 168 -177.

Davis, S. et al., "Effects of 60-Hz magnetic field exposure on nocturnal 6-sulfatoxymelatonin, estrogens, luteinizing hormone, & FSH in healthy reproductive-age women: results of a crossover trial. *Annals of Epidemiology*, Vol. 16 (8), 2006, p. 622–631

Draper, G. et al., "Childhood cancer in relation to distance from high voltage power lines in England and Wales: a case-control study." *BMJ*, Vol. 330, 2005, p. 1290-1294

Feigin, V. L. et al., "Solar & geomagnetic activities: are there associations with stroke occurrence?" *Cerebrovascular Diseases*, Vol. 7, 1997, p. 345–348

Gobba, F. et al., "Natural killer cell activity decreases in workers occupationally exposed to ELF magnetic fields exceeding 1 Micro T." *Int. J. Immunopathol. Pharmacol.*, Vol. 22, 2009, p. 1059-1066

Kay, R.W., "Geomagnetic storms: association with incidence of depression as measured by hospital admission." *British J. Psychiatry*, Vol. 164, 1994, p. 403–409

Levallois, P. et al., "Effects of electric & magnetic fields from high-power lines on female urinary excretion of 6- sulfatoxymelatonin." *Am. J. Epidemiol.*, Vol. 154 (7), 2001, p. 601–609

Linet. M. S. et al., "Residential exposure to magnetic fields & acute lymphoblastic leukemia in children." *NEJM.* Vol. 337 1997, p. 1-7

McKay, J. et al., "A literature review: the effects of magnetic field exposure on blood flow & blood vessels in the microvasculature." *BEMS*, Vol. 28, 2007, p. 81-98

Marino, A. et al., "Effect of low-frequency magnetic fields on brain electrical activity in human subjects." *Clinical Neurophysiology.* Vol. 115 (5), 2004, p. 1195-1201

Milham S. and E.M. Ossiander, "Historical evidence that residential electrification caused the emergence of the childhood leukemia peak." *Medical Hypothesis*, Vol. 56, 2001, p. 290-295.

O'Connor, R. P. and Persinger, M.A., "Geophysical variables & 93ulphate93: a strong association between SIDS & increments of global geomagnetic activity – possible support for the melatonin hypothesis." *Percept. Mo. Skills*, Vol. 84, 1997, p. 395–402

Okudan, B. et al., "DEXA analysis on the bones of rats exposed in utero and neonatally to static and 50 Hz electric fields." *Bioelectromagnetics*, Vol. 27, 2006, p. 589–592

Oraevskii, V.N., et al., "Medico-biological effect of natural electromagnetic variations". *Biofizika*, Vol. 43 (5), 1998, p. 844–888.

Patruno, A. et al., "ELF EMFs modulate expression of inducible nitric oxide synthase, endothelial NOS & cyclooxygenase-2 in the human keratinocyte cell line HaCat: potential therapeutic effects in wound healing." *British J. Dermatology.* Vol. 162 (2), 2010, p. 258-266

Persinger, M.A. and C. Psych, "Sudden unexpected death in epileptics following sudden, intense, increases in geomagnetic activity: prevalence of effect & potential mechanisms." Int. *J. Biometeorology*, Vol. 38, 1995, p. 180–187

Pfluger, D.H. and C.E. Minder, "Effects of exposure to 16.7 Hz magnetic fields on urinary 6-hydroxymelatonin 93sulphate excretion of Swiss railway workers." *J. Pineal Research*, Vol. 21, 1996, p. 91–100

Resch, J., "Geographic distribution of Multiple Sclerosis and comparison with geophysical values". *Soz Praventivmed*, Vol. 40 (3), 1995, p. 161–171.

Robertson, J. A. et al., "Low-frequency pulsed EMF exposure can alter neuroprocessing in humans." *J. R. Soc. Interfac*, Vol. 7, 2010, p. 467–473

Sakurai, T. et al., "Exposure to ELF magnetic fields affects insulin-secreting cells." *Bioelectromagnetics*, Vol. 29 (2), 2008, p. 118–124

Stoupel, E. et al., "Relationship between suicide & myocardial infarction with regard to changing physical environmental conditions." *Int. J. Biometeorol.*, Vol. 38, 1995, p. 199–203

Sliaupa, S., "Impact of some geological factors on human health." Proceedings of the International Seminar in Tamosava June 3–6, 2004

Tambiev, A.E., et al., "The effect of geomagnetic disturbances on the functions of attention and memory". *Aviakosm. Ekolog. Med.*, Vol. 29 (3), 1995, p. 43–45

[13] Meier, A., *A Worldwide Review of Standby Power Use in Homes.* Berkeley, CA: Lawrence Berkeley National Laboratory, 2002

Chapter 7 — Skin Contact Chemicals

[1] Mossman, S., *Fantastic Plastic Product & Design Consumer Culture.* Black Dog. 2008.

[2] Ibid.

[3] Mater, S and L. Hatch., *Chemistry of Petrochemical Processes.* 2nd Edition, Gulf Professional, ISBN 0884153150, 2001.

[4] Shafik, A. "Contraceptive efficacy of polyester-induced azoospermia in normal men." Contraception, Vol. 45 (5), 1992, p. 439–451

[5] Thornton, J., *Pandora's Poison; Chlorine, Health and a New Environmental Strategy.* Massachusetts Institute of Technology, 2000

[6] Vom Saal, F., {online] BPA References, [accessed Feb. 2011] http://endocrinedisruptors.missouri.edu/vomsaal/vomsaal.html

[7] Carlsen, E. et al., "Evidence for decreasing quality of semen during past 50 years." BMJ, Vol. 305, 1992, p. 609–613

[8] Maibach, H. I. et al., "Regional variation in percutaneous penetration in man." *Archives of Environmental Health,* Vol. 23, 1971, p.208–211

[9] Denda, M. and T. Tsuchiya, "Barrier recovery rate varies time-dependently in human skin." *Br. J. Dermatol.,* Vol. 142 (5), 2000, p. 881–884

[10] Benson, H.A.E. "assessment & clinical implications of absorption of sunscreens across skin." *Am. J. Clin. Dermatol.,* Vol. 1 (4), 2000, p. 217–224

[11] Lee, H. J. et al., "Antiandrogenic effects of BPA & nonylphenol on the function of androgen receptor." *Toxicol. Sci.,* Vol. 75, 2003, p. 40–46

[12] Ceccarelli, I. et al., "Estrogenic chemicals at puberty change ERalpha in the hypothalamus of male & female rats." *Neurotoxicol. Terato.,* Vol. 29, 2007, p.108–115

[13] Mendelsohn, M., [online] "Estrogens & cardiovascular disease." *European Congress of Endocrinology,* 2008. [Mar. 2009] www.Endocrine-Abstracts.Org/Ea/0016/Ea0016pl1.Htm

[14] Lovekamp-Swan, T. and B.J. Davis, "Mechanisms of phthalate ester toxicity in the female reproductive system." *EHP,* Vol. 111, 2003, p.139–145

Skakkebaek NE et al. "Testicular dysgenesis syndrome: an increasingly common developmental disorder with environmental aspects." *Human Reproduction,* Vol. 16, 2001, p. 972-978

[16] Huimin Y., "Exposure to BPA prenatally or in adulthood promotes th2 cytokine production associated with reduction of CD4+CD25+ regulatory T cells." *EHP,* Vol. 116 (4), 2008, p. 514–519

[17] Bushnik, T. et al., "Lead & BPA concentrations in the Canadian population." *Statcan.,* [accessed Nov. 2009] http://www.statcan.gc.ca/pub/82-003-x/2010003/article/11324-eng.pdf

[18] Bello, D. et al., "Skin exposure to isocyanates: reasons for concern." *EHP,* Vol. 115 (3), 2007, p. 328–335

[19] Hale, R.C. et al., "Potential role of fire retardant treated polyurethane foam as a source of brominated diphenyl ethers to the US environment." *Chemosphere,* Vol. 46, 2002, p. 729–735

[20] Ryan, J. and B. Patry, "Recent trends in levels of brominated diphenol ethers in human milks from Canada." *Organohalogen Compd,* Vol. 58, 2002, p. 173–176.

[21] Birnbaum, L. S. and D. F. Staskal., "Brominated flame retardants: cause for concern?" *EHP,* Vol. 112 (1), 2004, p. 9–17

[22] Mariussen, E. and F. Funnum., "The effect of pentabromodiphenyl ether, hexabromocyclododecaine and tetrabromobisphenol a on dopamine uptake into rat brain synaptosomes." *Organohalogen Compounds,* Vol. 57, 2002, p. 395–399

[23] Wiegand, H. et al., "Polyhalogenated hydrocarbon induced perturbation of intracellular calcium homeostasis; from astrocytes to human macrophages." *Organohalogen Compd.,* Vol. 53, 2001, p. 182–185

[24] Aydogan, M. et al., "The effect of vitamin C on BPA, nonylphenol & octylphenol induced brain damages of male rats." *Toxicol.,* Vol. 249, 2008, p. 35–39

Bindhumol, V., et al., "BPA induces reactive oxygen species generation in the liver of male rats." *Toxicology,* Vol. 188, 2003, p. 117–124

Chitra K.C. et al., "Induction of oxidative stress by BPA in the epididymal sperm of rats." *Toxicology*, Vol. 185 (1-2), 2003, p. 119–127

Chu, I. et al., "Skin reservoir formation & bioavailability of dermally administered chemicals in hairless guinea pigs." *Food Chem. Toxicol.*, Vol. 34, 1996, p. 267–276

Denda, M. and T. Tsuchiya, "Barrier recovery rate varies time-dependently in human skin." *British J. Dermatol.*, Vol. 142, 2000, p.881–884

Duty, S. et al., "Phthalate exposure & reproductive hormones in adult men." *Human Reproduction*, Vol. 20 (3), 2005, p. 604–610

Ema, M. et al., "Developmental effects of di-n-butyl phthalate after a single administration in rats." *J. App. Toxicology*, Vol. 17, 1997, p. 223–229

Fisher, J., "Environmental anti-androgens and male reproductive health: focus on phthalates and testicular dysgenesis syndrome." *Reproduction Update*, Vol. 127, 2004, p. 305–315.

Hauser, R, et al., "DNA damage in human sperm is related to urinary levels of phthalate monoester & oxidative metabolites." *Human Reproduction*, Vol. 22 (3), 2007, p. 688–695

Ho S.M. et al., "Developmental exposure to estradiol and BPA increases susceptibility to prostate carcinogenesis & epigenetically regulates phosphodiesterase." *Cancer Research*. Vol. 66, 2006, p. 5624–5632.

Huimin, Y. "Exposure to BPA prenatally or in adulthood promotes TH2 cytokine production associated with reduction of cd4+cd25+ regulatory T cells." *EHP*, Vol. 116 (4), 2008, p. 514–519

Kabuto, H. et al., "Exposure to BPA during embryonic/fetal life & infancy increases oxidative injury & causes underdevelopment of the brain and testis in mice." *Life Sciences*, Vol. 74, 2004, p. 2931–2940

Kanno, S. et al., "Effects of phytoestrogens & environmental estrogens on osteoblastic differentiation in MC3T3-E1 cells." *Toxicol.*, Vol. 196, 2004, p. 137–145

Krone, C. A. et al., "Isocyanates in flexible polyurethane foams." *Environmental Contamination and Toxicology*, Vol. 70 (2), 2003, p. 328–335

Lang, I. A. et al., "Association of urinary BPA concentration with medical disorders and laboratory abnormalities in adults: evidence from NHANES 2003/4." *JAMA*, Vol. 300 (11), 2008, p. 1303-1310

Meeker, J et al., "Urinary BPA concentrations in relation to serum thyroid and reproductive hormones in men from an infertility clinic" *Environmental Science & Technology*. Vol. 44 (4), 2010, p. 1458–1463

Ropero, A. B. et al., "BPA disruption of the endocrine pancreas & blood glucose homeostasis." *International J. Andrology*, Vol. 31, 2008, p. 194-200

Segura, J. J. et al., "In vitro effect of the resin component BPA on substrate adherence capacity of macrophages." *J. Endodontics*, Vol. 25, 1999, p. 341–344

Stahlhut, R. W. et al., "Concentrations of urinary phthalate metabolites are associated with increased waist circumference & insulin resistance in adult U.S. males." *EHP*, Vol. 115 (6), 2007, p. 876–882

Swan, S. H. et al., "Decrease in anogenital distance among male infants with prenatal phthalate exposure." *EHP*, Vol. 113 (8), 2005, p. 1056–1061

Takeuchi, T., "Positive relationship between androgen & the endocrine disruptor, BPA, in normal women & women with ovarian dysfunction." *Endocr. J.*, Vol. 51 (2), 2004, p. 165–169

Tokura, H. et al., "Mechanism of pyjama material on stratum corneum water content under mild cold conditions: explored by hierarchical linear regression." *Skin Research & Technology*, Vol. 13 (4), 2007, p. 412–416

Trevillian, L. F. et al., "Infant sleeping environment & asthma at 7 years." *Am. J. Public Health*, Vol. 95, 2005, p. 2238–2245

Vom Saal, F.S., "Low-Dose BPA: confirmed by an extensive literature." *Chemistry &Industry*, Vol. 7, 2005, p. 14–15

Weigand, H. et al., "Polyhalogenated hydrocarbon induced perturbation of intracellular calcium homeostasis; from astrocytes to human macrophages." *Organohalogen Compounds*, Vol. 53, 2001, p. 182-185

Wetherill, Y.B., et al. "The xenoestrogen BPA induces inappropriate androgen receptor activation & mitogenesis in prostate adeno-carcinoma cells." *Molecular Cancer Therapeutics*, Vol. 7, 2002, p. 515–524

Chapter 8 — Air Pollutants

[1] Dethlefsen, U. and R. Repgas., "A new therapy for nighttime asthma" "(Ein neues therapieprinzip bei nachtlichen asthma)." *Klinicheskaia Meditsina*, Vol. 80, 1985, p. 44–7

[2] Bushnell, P. J. et al., "Effects of toluene inhalation on detection of auditory signals in rats." *Neurotoxic. & Teratol.* Vol. 16 (2), 1994, p. 149–160

Yamamoto, S. et al., "Children's immunology, what can we learn from animal studies." *J. Toxicological Sciences*, Vol. 34, 2009, p. 341–348

[3] Hirvonen, M. et al., "Effect of growth medium on potential of Streptomyces anulatus spores to induce inflammatory responses & cytotoxicity in macrophages." *Inhalation Toxicology*, Vol. 13, 2001, p. 55–68

[4] Swan, W., "Atmospheric electricity & ionization." *Proceedings of International Conference of Ionization of the Air*, Vol. 2, 1961, p. 1–16

[5] Rosenberg, B., "A study of atmospheric ionization: measurements of the ion conditions in an ATC laboratory & literature review", *National Aviation Facilities Experimental Center*, Report No. NA-72-19, May 1972.

Nagy, R., "Nature of air ions generated by different methods", *Proceedings of Int. Conference of Ionization of the Air*, Vol. 1, 1961, p. 1–13

[6] Kreuger, P. A. and S. Kotaka., "The effect of air ions on brain levels of seratonin in mice." *International J. Biometeorology*, Vol. 13, 1969, p. 25–38

[7] Pratt, R. and R. Barnard., "Some effects of ionized air on Penicillium notatum." *J. Am. Pharmaceutical Association*, Vol. 49, 1960, p. 643–646.

Furst, R., "Studies on ionization effects." *Annual Report*. Houston , Anderson Hospital, Houston University of Texas. 1955

Phillips, G. et al., "Effects of air ions on bacterial aerosols." *Int. J. Biometeorol*, Vol. 8, 1964, p. 27–37

Kellogg, E. et al., "Superoxide involvement in the bactericidal effects of negative ions on Staphylococcus albus." *Nature*, Vol. 281, 1979, p. 400-401

Shargawi, J., et al., "Sensitivity of Candida Albicans to negative air ion streams." *J. Applied Microbiology*, Vol. 87 (6), 1999, p. 889-897

Noyce, J., et al., "Bactericidal effects of negative & positive ions generated in nitrogen on E-Coli." *J. Electrostatics*, Vol. 54, 2002, p. 179-187

[8] Shepherd S. et al., "Effect of negative air ions on the potential for bacterial contamination of plastic medical equipment." *BMC Infect. Dis.*, Vol. 10, 2010, p.92

[9] Strahil, T. et al., "The relationship between sleep & asthma." *Sleep Med. Clin.*, Vol. 2, 2007, p. 9–18

[10] Akingbemi B. T. et al."Phthalate-induced leydig cell hyperplasia is associated with multiple endocrine disturbances." *Proc. Natl. Acad. Sci.* Vol. 101 (3), 2004, p. 775-780

Alonso-Magdalena, P. et al., "The estrogenic effect of BPA disrupts the pancreatic beta cell function in vivo and induces insulin resistance." *EHP*, Vol. 114, 2006, p. 106-112

Bornehag, C.G. et al., "The association between asthma & allergic symptoms in children & phthalates in house dust: a nested case-control study." *EHP*, Vol. 112, 2004, p. 1393-1397

Bräuner, E.V. et al., "Indoor particles affect vascular function in the aged: an air filtration-based intervention study." *Am. J. Respir. Crit. Care Med.*, Vol. 177, 2008, p. 419-425

Ceccarelli, I. et al., "Estrogenic chemicals at puberty change ERalpha in the hypothalamus of male & female rats." *Neurobehavioral Toxicology & Teratology,* Vol. 29 (1), 2007, p. 108–115

Daniels, S. L., "On the ionization of air for removal of noxious effluvia", *IEEE Transactions on Plasma Science,* Vol. 30, 2002, p. 1471–1481

Dodge, J.A., "Environmental estrogens: effects on cholesterol lowering and bone in the ovariectomized rat." *J. Steroid Biochem. Mol. Biol.,* Vol. 59, 1996, p. 155–161

Feige, J. N. et al., "The pollutant diethylhexyl phthalate regulates hepatic energy metabolism via species-specific PPAR[Alpha]-dependent mechanisms." *EHP,* Vol. 118 (2), 2010, p. 234

Franklin, P. et al., "Raised exhaled nitric oxide in healthy children is associated with domestic formaldehyde levels." *Am. J. Respir. Crit. Care Med.,* Vol. 161, 2000, p. 1757–1759

Freire, C. et al., "Association of traffic-related air pollution with cognitive development in children." *JECH*, Vol. 64 (3), 2010, p. 223–228

Furst, R., "Studies on ionization effects." *Annual Report.* Houston , Anderson Hospital, Houston University of Texas. 1955

Grabarczyk. Z., "Effectiveness of indoor air cleaning with corona ionizers", *J. Electrostatics*, Vol. 51–52, 2001, p. 278–283

Gurel, A. et al., "Vitamin E against oxidative damage caused by formaldehyde in frontal cortex and hippocampus: biochemical & histological studies." *J. Chemical Neuroanatomy,* Vol. 29, 2005, p. 173–178

Kellogg, E. et al., "Superoxide involvement in the bactericidal effects of negative ions on staphylococcus albus." *Nature*, Vol. 281, 1979, p. 400–401.

Kim, Y.S. et al., "Application of air ions for bacterial de-colonization in air filters contaminated by aerosolized bacteria." *Sci. Total Environ.*, Vol. 409(4), 2011, p. 748–755

Kolarik, B., "The association between phthalates in dust and allergic diseases among Bulgarian children." *EHP*, Vol. 116 (1), 2008, p. 98–103

Lagercrantz, L. et al., "Nitric Oxide in exhaled & aspirated nasal air as an objective measure of human response to isopropanol oxidation products & phthalate esters." *10th International Conference on IAQ & Climate,* Vol. 5, 2005, p. 3855–3858. Beijing: Tsinghua University Press

Lang, I.A. et al., "Association of urinary BPA concentration with medical disorders & laboratory abnormalities in adults: evidence from NHANES 2003/4." *JAMA*, Vol. 300 (11), 2008, p. 1303-1310

Lee, B.U. et al., "Removal of fine & ultrafine particles from indoor air environments by unipolar ion emission", *Atmospheric Environment*, Vol. 38, 2004, p. 4815–4823

Loh, M.M. et al., "Ranking cancer risks of organic hazardous air pollutants in the US." *EHP*, Vol. 115 (8), 2007, p. 1160–1168

Noyce, J. et al., "Bactericidal effects of negative & positive ions generated in nitrogen on E-Coli." *J. Electrostatics*, Vol. 54, 2002, p. 179–187

Phillips, G. et al., "Effects of air ions on bacterial aerosols." *Int. J. Biometeorol.*, Vol. 8, 1964, p. 27–37.

Pratt, R. and R. Barnard., "Some effects of ionized air on Penicillium Notatum." *J. Am. Pharmaceutical Association*, Vol. 49, 1960, p. 643–646.

Reilly, T. and I. C. Stevenson., "An investigation of the effects of negative air ions on responses to submaximal exercise at different times of day." *JHE*, Vol. 22 (1), 1993, p. 1–9

Sax, L., *Boys Adrift: The Five Factors Driving the Growing Epidemic of Unmotivated Boys and Underachieving Young Men*. Basic Books. 2007

Shargawi, J. et al., "Sensitivity of Candida Albicans to negative air ion streams." *J. Applied Microbiology*, Vol. 87 (6), 1999, p. 889–897

Sherriff, A. et al., "Frequent use of chemical household products is associated with persistent wheezing in pre-school children." *Thorax*, Vol. 60, 2005, p. 45–49

Turner M. C. et al., "Residential pesticides & childhood leukemia: a systematic review and meta-analysis." *EHP*, Vol. 118 (1) 2010, p. 33–41

Wang T. et al., "Particulate matter disrupts human lung endothelial barrier integrity via ROS- and p38 MAPK-dependent pathways." *Am. J. Respir. Cell Mol. Biol.*, Vol. 42, 2010, p. 442–449

[11] National Aeronautics & Space Administration. *Interior Landscape Plants for Indoor Air Pollution Abatement*. September 15, 1989

[12] Alonso, J.M. and J.R. Ecker. "The ethylene pathway: a paradigm for plant hormone signalling & interaction." *Science's STK : Signal Transduction Knowledge Environment*, Vol. 95 (6), 2001, p. 901–915

[13] Ulrich, M.M., "Health effects & time course of particulate matter on the cardiopulmonary system in rats with lung inflammation." *J. Toxicol. Environ. Health*, Vol. 65, 2002, p. 1571–1595

[14] Pope, C. A. et al., "Lung cancer, cardiopulmonary mortality, & long-term exposure to fine particulate air pollution." *JAMA*, Vol. 287 (9), 2002, p. 1132–1141

Index

About the Author

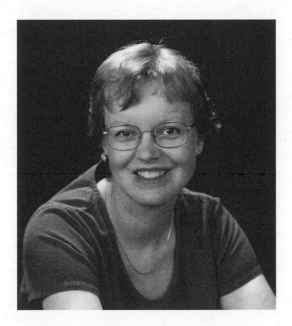

Angela Hobbs was herself once a victim of chemicals, electrical, and location specific sensitivities. After using research skills, gleaned from a career in management consulting, to find her own solutions, she shared her story in The Sick House Survival Guide: Simple Steps to Healthier Homes (New Society 2003). Since then a flood of inquiries from all over the world have taken Hobbs on a research-powered journey of discovery that resulted in her growing insight into the multi-faceted mechanisms by which location can influence our sleep mechanisms to the detriment of our health.

Hobbs is now a wellness consultant delivering personal and commercial programs that assess bedrooms, educate people about the steps they can take to improve their sleep, and help corporations increase workforce productivity. She lives with her husband and two sons near Calgary, Alberta, Canada.